Practical Hints
To
CLINICAL
ELECTROCARDIOGRAPHY

Practical Hints To CLINICAL ELECTROCARDIOGRAPHY

C R Maiti MD (Cal), FRCP (Glassgow), DTM (Cal)
Professor of Medicine and Head, Department of Cardiology (Retd.),
Medical College, Kolkata

N Goswami MBBS (Cal)

New Central Book Agency (P) Ltd
LONDON
DELHI KOLKATA PUNE HYDERABAD ERNAKULAM

REGD OFFICE
8/1 Chintamoni Das Lane, Kolkata 700 009, India
email: ncbapvtltd@eth.net

OVERSEAS
NCBA (UK) Ltd, 149 Park Avenue North, Northampton, NN3 2HY, UK

EXPORT
NCBA Exports Pvt. Ltd, 212 Shahpur Jat, New Delhi 110 049
email: ncbaexp@ncbapvtltd.com

BRANCHES

208B Peacock Lane, Shahpur Jat
New Delhi 110 049
email: ncbadel@ncbapvtltd.com

Shop Nos. 3 & 4, Vinayak Towers
681/B Budhwar Peth, Appa Balwant Chowk
Pune 411 002
email: ncbapune@ncbapvtltd.com

House No. 3-1-315, 1st Floor
Nimboliadda, Kachiguda, **Hyderabad** 500 027
email: ncbahydb@ncbapvtltd.com

GSS Shopping Complex, 1st Floor
Opposite College Post Office, Convent Road
Ernakulam 682 035
email: ncbaernk@ncbapvtltd.com

PRACTICAL HINTS TO CLINICAL ELECTROCARDIOGRAPHY

First Published: January 1973
Reprinted with Additions: June 1977
Second Edition: September 1986
Reprinted with Additions: June 1995
Reprinted: January 1999
Thoroughly Revised Third Edition: October 2002
Reprinted: January 2009, Reprinted: January 2011

PUBLISHER AND TYPESETTER
New Central Book Agency (P) Ltd
8/1 Chintamoni Das Lane, Kolkata 700 009

PRINTER
New Central Book Agency (P) Ltd
Web-Offset Division, Dhulagarh, Sankrail, Howrah

COVER PRINTER
Biswanath Studio, Kolkata

PROJECT SUPERVISOR
Subas Maitra

PROJECT TEAM
Himangshu Acharya, Tarun Dey, and Prabhat Jas

ISBN: 81-7381-106-7

Price: ₹ 250.00

Dedicated

To

Lovers of Medicine

FOREWORD

The small monograph **Practical Hints to Clinical Electrocardiography** by Dr. C. R. Maiti, M.D., M.R.C.P., D.T.M. and Dr. N. Goswami, M.B.B.S. of the Heart Unit, Medical College and Hospital, Calcutta, contains selected electrocardiograms, illustrative of the different cardiac arrhythmias, conduction defects and various types of heart diseases. The description of the electrocardiograms is concise and to the point without any reference to the complex theories of electrocardiography. It is hoped this monograph would help the senior medical students and the busy medical practitioners to acquire a practical knowledge of clinical electrocardiography which will be useful aid in the diagnosis of the diseases of the heart.

The authors deserve our appreciation for the contribution to the existing store of books on Clinical Electrocardiography.

Calcutta
28th November
1972

J. C. Banerjea
M.B. (Cal.), F.R.C.P. (Lond.)

Publisher's Note to the Revised Third Edition

This book is unique of its kind. It gives not only PRACTICAL HINTS but also substantiates them with enough theory to back them up. And, the author has taken immense pains in edition after edition to incorporate the latest and modern interpretations of ELECTROCARDIOGRAM.

In this updated and revised Third Edition, too, the author has added a valuable chapter **CARDIAC PACING AND ELECTROCARDIOGRAM.** Therein latest patterns of ECG tracings in different types of artificial pacemakers are clearly illustrated to give the readers a clear grasp of this life-saving system.

For these very reasons this monograph has enjoyed the confidence of discerning students and the patronage of their erudite professors for the last 30 years. And we would consider it our ample reward if we can be of such service to them in future too.

DR. MITA SEN
M.B.B.S.

PREFACE TO THE SECOND EDITION

The book was exhausted a long time ago. Since then, there has been a persistent demand of this book by the students which has prompted me to bring out a thoroughly revised second edition within a possible compass of time.

In this edition, some newer topics such as 'electrophysiology of heart', 'His bundle electrocardiography', and 'Recent methods of electrocardiography' have been discussed with illustrative diagrams. This would, I trust, help the beginners to have a clearer concept of the basis and interpretation of electrocardiogram.

I am grateful to all my colleagues, friends and senior students for their kind suggestions in bringing out this edition.

N. Goswami, my co-author, had permanently joined Ramakrishna Mission Ashram, Belur Math, Howrah, for which he was not able to make further contribution towards the subsequent additions or editions. I deeply regret his loss.

My grateful thanks are also due to the publishers for their kind assistance, without which this edition would not have seen the light of the day.

September 1986 **C. R. Maiti**

PREFACE TO THE FIRST EDITION

A manifold increase in the incidence of heart disease has taken place in recent years. There has been an explosion in the field of ischaemic heart disease which has practically spared no age and no sex in recent times. Hurry and worry, anxiety and tension, specially of urban life, dietary indiscretion, inadequate rest, overcrowding population, infections, increased longevity, etc., have all contributed towards the tremendous increase in the incidence of heart disease.

Electrocardiogram is an indispensable aid for different cardiac conditions and no opinion can be given on heart cases without it. It is one of the essential methods of investigations in the practice of medicine. It is required for the diagnosis of heart disease, for exclusion of heart disease, as a preparatory investigation for operations, specially in advanced age, to follow up cases of heart disease, for medical check up, etc. The investigation is so easy and simple that it is accepted by any patient.

It was a dream for us to write a book on electrocardiogram, although we had felt the need of such a book for a long time. Our students demanded a simple and easy interpretation of electrocardiogram which has been rendered relatively difficult in most books for ordinary students of medicine. It had been our constant worry how to make things easy for students. This was the impetus which forced us to write such a book.

The book is not meant for the masters of medicine. This would only help the beginners of average calibre and give them impetus to learn further. The book has been written with the purpose of imparting basic concepts of electrocardiogram in a concise manner to the new entrants on the subject. Such a book must of necessity have its limitations and we have intentionally omitted the technical details, names of authors and workers and references, to make things easy and simple. A clinical approach to the subject has been made and it is expected that this would help the clinicians.

We are grateful to Dr. Subrata Gupta and Dr. Arjun Gupta who encouraged us to write this book. We are indebted to Dr. Harendra Nath Chatterjee and Dr. Debiprosad Chatterjee for their ungrudging help and encouragement to prepare this monograph.

We are indebted to Prof. J. C. Banerjea for revision of this monograph and writing a foreword for this book.

Our grateful thanks are also due to Dr. Sunil Kar, Dr. J. P. Baral, Dr. Anil Saha, Dr. Banikantha Das Sarkar and Mr. J. M. Chatterjee for their valuable assistance in bringing out this book.

We are also grateful to the publishers for their kind suggestions and assistance without which it would have been impossible to publish this book.

Calcutta
5th December
1972

C. R. Maiti
N. Goswami

CONTENTS

CHAPTER I

INTRODUCTION

Definition of an electrocardiogram

An electrocardiogram is a graphic representation of the electrical activity (depolarisation and repolarisation) of the heart.

Basic principles

Various waves in the electrocardiogram are produced by the flow of electricity towards or away from the electrodes which are routinely placed over the surface of the body.

When electricity flows towards the electrode, the deflection of the stylus of the electrocardiograph machine is upwards, i.e., positive.

When the electricity flows away from the electrode the deflection of the stylus is downwards, i.e., negative.

When there is no flow of electricity, there is no deflection and an iso-electric base line is drawn across the tracing paper.

Various leads

Leads are patterns of arrangement of electrodes placed on different areas of the body surface to study the electrical activity of the heart by means of deflections in the galvanometer of the electrocardiograph.

Leads may be Bipolar or Unipolar.

Bipolar leads

These show the potential difference between two areas over the body surface. There are bipolar standard leads and bipolar chest leads.

Bipolar standard leads

In these, the electrodes are placed on two different limbs of the body. These are:

Lead I—Connects right arm and left arm.
Lead II—Connects right arm and left leg.
Lead III—Connects left arm and left leg.

Bipolar chest leads

These are named CR, CL and CF leads. Here the so-called indifferent electrode is placed on the right arm, left arm, and left leg in case of CR, CL and CF leads respectively and the exploring electrode is placed on the chest wall from V_1 to V_6 position and onward and is designated as CR_1, CL_1, CF_1, CR_2, CL_2, CF_2, etc. These leads are not helpful as it is now realised that the small potential that may be present in the extremities may alter the pattern of the electrocardiogram obtained from chest leads.

Unipolar leads

These show the actual potential over an area on the body surface; two electrodes are used; the electrode used to detect the actual potential over a particular point on the body surface is called the exploring electrode, the other one being the indifferent electrode recording no potential. There are unipolar limb leads and unipolar chest leads.

Unipolar limb leads (augmented voltage leads)

There are 3 unipolar limb leads—aVR, aVL, aVF; here the exploring electrode is placed over the right arm, left arm and left foot respectively.

aVR—shows potential in the right arm.

aVL—shows potential in the left arm.

aVF—shows potential in the left leg.

Unipolar chest leads (voltage leads)

In case of unipolar chest leads the exploring electrode is placed in different areas over the chest wall. These leads are named according to the position of the exploring electrode and they are as follows:

V_1—Over the lateral sternal line in the right 4th intercostal space.

V_2—Over the lateral sternal line in the left 4th intercostal space.

V_3—In the midpoint between V_2 and V_4 positions.

V_4—In the left 5th intercostal space in the midclavicular line.

V_5—In the horizontal level of V_4 lead in the left anterior axillary line.

V_6—In the horizontal level of V_4 lead in the left midaxillary line.

V_7—In the horizontal level of V_4 lead in the left posterior axillary line.

V_8—In the horizontal level of V_4 lead in the left scapular line.

V_9—In the horizontal level of V_4 lead in the left border of the spine.

When the exploring electrode for V (chest) leads are placed on the right side of the chest instead of on the left side they are designated as V_3R, V_4R, V_5R lead, etc. The V_E lead is the unipolar chest lead where the exploring electrode is placed over the ensiform cartilage.

$3V_{1-9}$ represents V leads taken one intercostal space higher i.e. $3V_{1-9}$ indicates V_{1-9} leads taken from the level of 3rd left intercostal space. Thus similar terminology can be applied when V_{1-9} leads are taken from the level of 2nd ($2V_{1-9}$) and 6th ($6V_{1-9}$) left intercostal spaces. If Ecg. is taken similarly from the right side the term $3V_{3-9}$R may be used.

Monitor leads

In a coronary care unit, a modified bipolar chest lead (monitor lead) is used for constant observations of the pattern of Ecg. of the cardiac patient.

Here the positive electrode is placed in the V_1 position, the negative electrode near the left shoulder and a third electrode is placed at a more distant point over the chest say, just below the right clavicle which serves as a ground electrode. The pattern of Ecg. in this lead is almost similar to V_1 lead. ST-T wave changes in the Ecg. due to myocardial ischaemia or due to variation in the serum potassium level may be seen better when the positive electrode is placed in the V_4 or V_5 position in the monitor lead.

Classically a 12-lead electrocardiogram is done taking the tracing in the following leads: standard leads I, II, III, unipolar limb leads aVR, aVL, aVF and unipolar chest leads from V_1 to V_6.

Esophageal lead (E lead)

In this case the exploring electrode is passed through the nares into the oesophagus of the patient and its exact position is determined by screening; it may be placed above, below or at the level of the heart. It helps to record the left atrial events and explore the postero-inferior surface of the left ventricle more distinctly than any classical lead.

Intracardiac lead

The electrocardiogram may be recorded with the exploring electrode inside cardiac chambers and great vessels by means of a special lead called intracardiac lead. The lead is introduced through a systemic vein usually through the median cubital or the internal jugular vein into the right atrium and other chambers of the heart, and the great vessels with the help of screening. Inside the different chambers of the heart and the great vessels characteristic tracings are obtained. The intracavity lead is applied for guidance and detection of the exact position of the tip of the cardiac catheter during catheter studies by noting the characteristic tracing (Fig. 1).

(a)

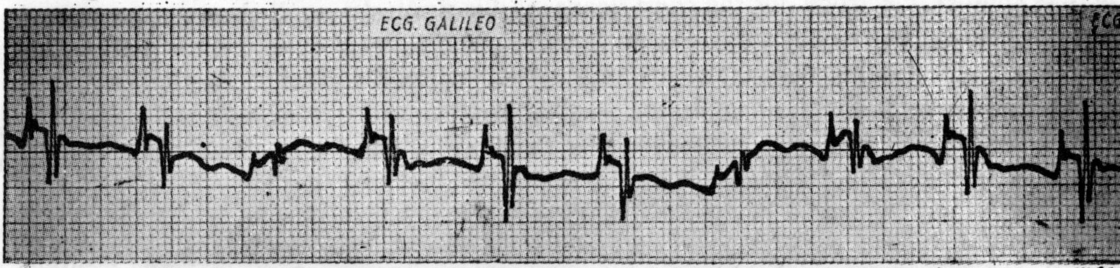

(b)

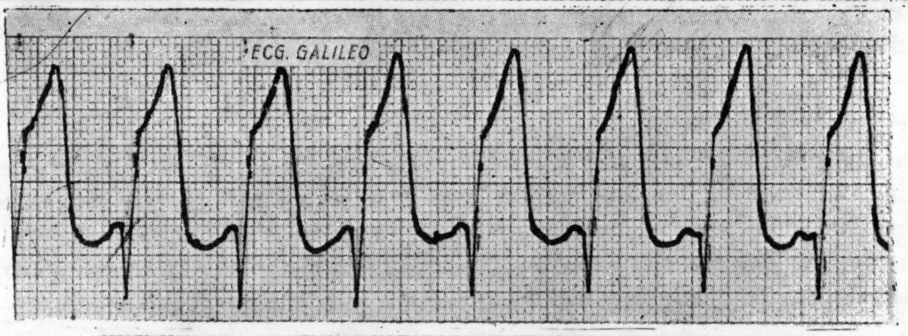

(c)

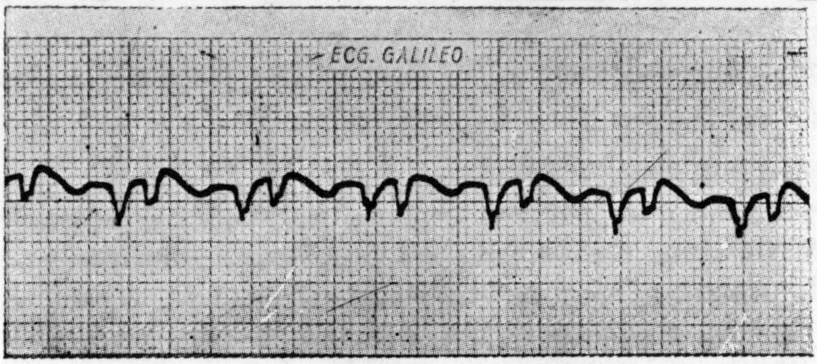

Fig. 1. An intracardiac electrocardiogram.

Fig. 1(a) is a tracing from coronary sinus. Fig. 1(b) is a tracing from the cavity of right ventricle. Fig. 1(c) is a tracing from inside the right atrium.

The electrocardiograph

It is a highly sensitive moving-coil galvanometer which records the passage of electricity and voltage difference between two points on the body surface. The galvanometer deflection is observed from the movement of a heated stylus which causes inscriptions on the electrocardiograph paper running at a uniform speed with the help of a motor. The different leads are selected by means of a lead selector. One end of the patient's cable is fixed to the body surface of the patient by electrodes fixed by rubber straps with a conducting material intervening between the skin and the electrodes and the other end of the cable is fixed to the machine by a suitable adaptor.

The electrocardiograph paper

It is a specially prepared graph paper on which small squares of absolutely uniform size are drawn. The breadth of each small square represents 0·04 sec. when the tracing paper runs at a speed of 25 mm. per sec.; the height of each small square represents 0·1 millivolt after usual standardisation and is designated as 1 mm.

The technique of recording electrocardiogram

The person is preferably placed in the supine position. The electrodes are applied firmly with rubber straps around each limb after rubbing the skin with electrocardiographic jelly (a preparation of sodium chloride) for better conduction of electricity. There is another electrode for the chest leads and is similarly applied over the skin of the chest wall. The input channels of the patient's cable are connected to the electrodes fixed at different sites over the body surface as per labels on the cable.

The other end of the input channels of the patient's cable is socketted into the machine through a specially designed adaptor. The machine is then connected with the mains through a mains cable. The machine is then switched on. By rotating the sensitivity control knob the deflection of the heated stylus is controlled in such a way that it gives a deflection of 10 mm. for 1 millivolt. The lead selector is then put in a lead position in which the electrocardiogram is to be taken. The deflections of the heated stylus are then noticed and as soon as the deflections are found to be steady the tracing paper is run for recording.

Utility of doing an electrocardiogram

With the advent of exercise electrocardiograms (eg. treadmill test), Holter technique of Ecg. recording, teletransmission and recording of Ecg., echocardiography etc., a resting Ecg. is only of a limited value. As the present book only deals with the techniques and interpretations of a resting Ecg., readers should consult special monographs for Holter monitoring system, teletransmission and tape recording of Ecg., treadmill tests etc.

An Ecg. is of particular value in the following conditions.

(1) To diagnose myocardial infarction, coronary insufficiency and angina pectoris.

(2) To detect various types of cardiac arrhythmias.

(3) To get evidences of pericarditis.

(4) To observe myocardial changes accompanying pericarditis, myo-pericarditis, myxœdema, after intake of drugs, connective tissue diseases, disturbances by an abnormal electrolyte metabolism. etc.

(5) To detect conduction defects and heart block.

(6) To recognise enlargement of atria and ventricles.

CHAPTER II

ELECTROPHYSIOLOGY OF HEART

Genesis of an electrocardiogram

The genesis of an electrocardiogram involves the following steps.

(1) In the sinus node there is formation of an impulse or initiation of a wave of excitation.

(2) The impulse which originates in the sinus node begins to travel through a specialised tissue following a definite path.

(3) As soon as the impulse reaches the atrial and ventricular muscles there is activation (depolarisation) and contraction of these muscles.

(4) Soon after depolarisation a process of recovery or repolarisation starts.

(5) The process of depolarisation and repolarisation generates a flow of electricity.

Cellular potentials

If one electrode is placed over one point of a resting muscle cell and another electrode is placed over another point over the same resting muscle cell away from the first one, there will be no flow of electricity due to zero potential.

If the surface membrane of the muscle cell is penetrated by a capillary electrode, there will be a flow of electricity due to development of a negative potential. This is called 'membrane resting potential'.

A high concentration of intracellular potassium ions and a low concentration of potassium ions outside the cells result in a gradient of potassium ions across the cell membrane to the extent of about 30:1. This is mainly responsible for the development of a negative potential and the flow of electricity.

The cell membrane is much more permeable to potassium ions than to sodium ions in its resting state.

The entry and exit of sodium ions through the muscle cell membrane is said to be an active process and is called 'the sodium pump' and is believed to provide the source of energy for a high concentration of potassium ions inside the cells.

The cell membrane is much less permeable to sodium ions than potassium ions in its resting state. A high concentration of potassium ions inside the cells and the negative membrane resting potential are believed to be derived from energy obtained from the active transport of sodium ions into the cells.

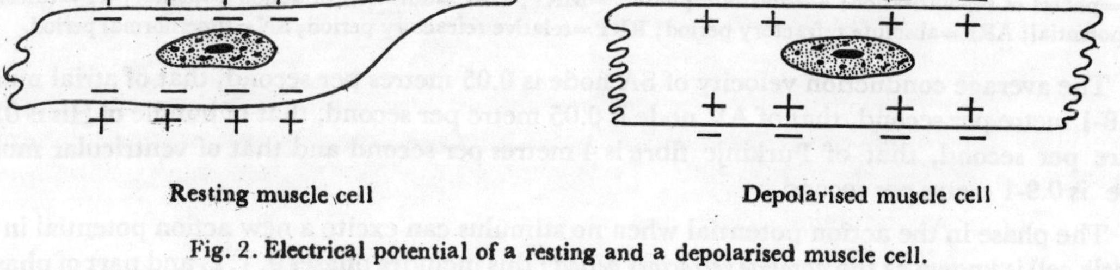

Fig. 2. Electrical potential of a resting and a depolarised muscle cell.

The permeability of cell membrane alters with the onset of depolarisation of a muscle cell. The entry of sodium ions into the cells causes a sharp rise of intracellular potential to positivity (approximately 20mV). This initial phase of depolarisation is known as phase O. Following this initial quick phase the intracellular potential gradually returns to the membrane resting potential. This phase of repolarisation is usually divided into 4 phases: Phase 1 where there is an initial rapid phase of repolarisation, phase 2 where there is a plateau period because of a slow process of repolarisation, phase 3 where there is a residual gradual return of the intracellular potential towards the resting potential, and phase 4, when the intracellular potential actually reaches the membrane resting potential.

The "Sodium pump" operates with extrusion of sodium from the cells during the process of repolarisation. During phases 1 and 2 potassium goes out of the cell and during phase 3 potassium ions get inside the cell with restoration of membrane resting potential. The duration from the onset of depolarisation to the termination of repolarisation is the duration of the action potential.

The action potential curve of a cell in the sino-atrial node is different from that of a ventricular or atrial muscle cell by a lower membrane resting potential at the onset of diastole, a gradual rise of the membrane resting potential during the phase of diastole, a slow depolarisation, a rounded peak of the action potential and a slow single curve of repolarisation where the phases 1, 2, and 3 cannot be defined.

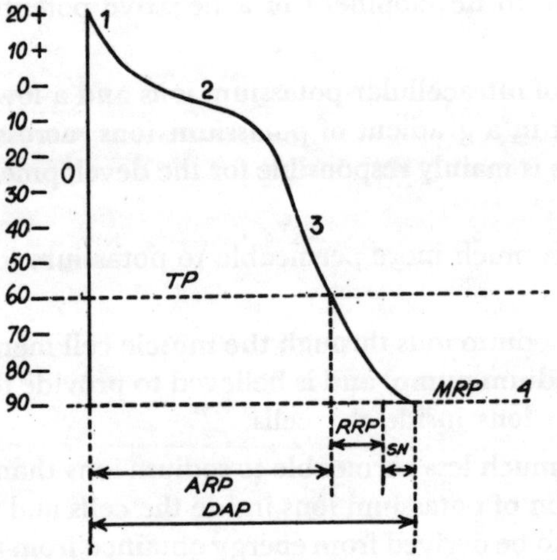

Fig 3. Diagram of action potential of a ventricular muscle cell; MRP=membrane resting potential; 1, 2, and 3 =phases of repolarisation; 4=diastolic phase =MRP; DAP=duration of action potential; TP=threshold potential; ARP=absolute refractory period; RRP=relative refractory period; SN=supernormal period.

The average conduction velocity of SA node is 0.05 metres per second, that of atrial muscle is 0.8-1 metre per second, that of AV node is 0.05 metre per second, that of bundle of His is 0.8-1 metre per second, that of Purkinje fibre is 4 metres per second and that of ventricular muscle fibre is 0.9-1 metre per second.

The phase in the action potential when no stimulus can excite a new action potential in the muscle cell is known as the ***absolute refractory period;*** this includes phases 0, 1, 2, and part of phase 3.

Following the phase of absolute refractory period, a strong stimulus may evoke a response; this is *relative refractory period* which begins when the transmembrane potential in phase 3 reaches the threshold potential level. This is again followed by a *phase of supernormal excitability* during which a weak stimulus can evoke a response; it is found in terminal part of phase 3 and beginning of phase 4.

Electrical potentials of a normal muscle cell

The entire surface of a muscle cell has zero potential due to high impedance of the cell membrane.

When an isolated strip of muscle is stimulated, the surface of the stimulated part of the muscle strip becomes electrically negative which advances progressively; the surface of the muscle strip not stimulated remains electrically positive. (Fig. 4.)

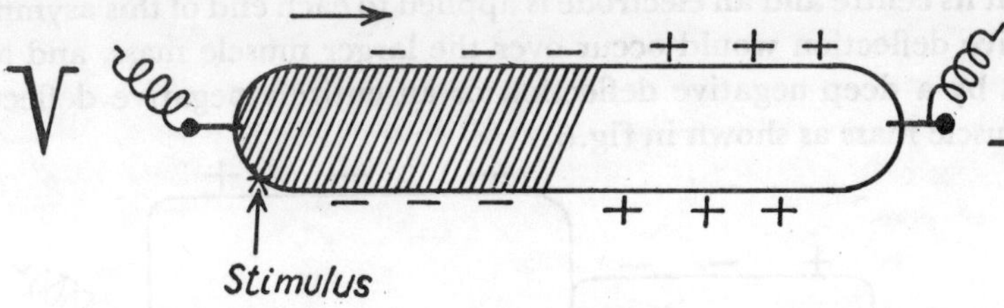

Fig. 4. Electrical potential of a stimulated muscle strip.

Depolarisation: Initial depolarisation is the initial spread of the stimulus through the muscle strip. The upward or downward deflection of the tracing depends on the direction of spread of the stimulus and the exact position of the electrode applied to the muscle strip.

The deflection of the stylus will be upwards if the stimulus *spreads towards* the electrode. The deflection will be downwards if the stimulus *spreads away* from the concerned electrode. If the electrode is applied to the middle of the muscle strip the deflection will be diphasic as the current flows from one end to the other end of the strip.

If the electrode is placed in the middle of the muscle strip and the stimulus is given at its one end there would be a diphasic deflection, the initial deflection being upward due to the advancing positive charge and the second deflection being downward due to the flowing of this negative charge. (Fig. 4a)

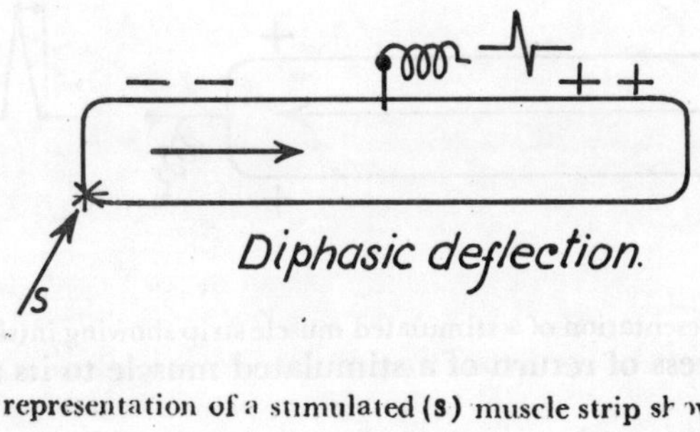

Fig. 4a. A diagrammatic representation of a stimulated (S) muscle strip showing diphasic deflection.

Now, if a muscle strip is stimulated in its middle the excitation wave spreads simultaneously towards both ends of the muscle strip and if an electrode is applied to each end of the muscle strip, a positive or upward deflection of depolarisation of equal magnitude would occur at either end. (Fig. 5)

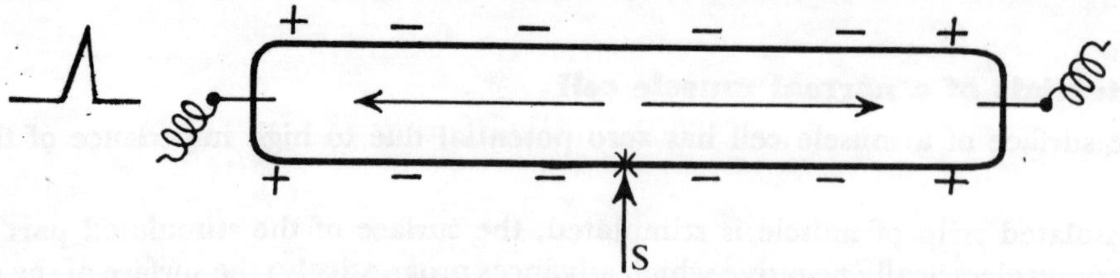

Fig. 5. A muscle strip stimulated(s) at its centre.

If the muscle mass is asymmetrical, one side being bigger than the other and the said muscle strip is stimulated at its centre and an electrode is applied to each end of this asymmetrical muscle strip, a large positive deflection would occur over the larger muscle mass, and a small positive deflection followed by a deep negative deflection or an entirely negative deflection will occur over the smaller muscle mass as shown in fig. 6.

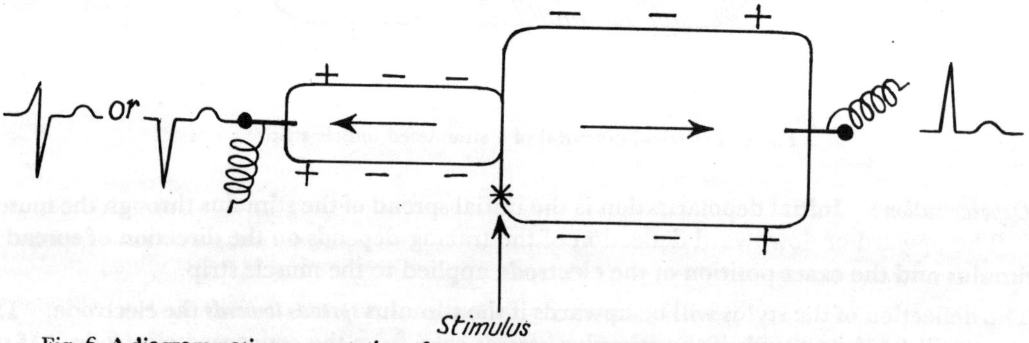

Fig. 6. A diagrammatic representation of an asymmetrical muscle mass with galvanometric deflections when electrodes are applied at each end of the strip after stimulation (vide text).

Intrinsic deflection: The intrinsic (or intrinsicoid) deflection time or ventricular activation time (VAT) is the time required for the spread of the impulse from one end to the other end of the muscle strip and is calculated by measuring the interval from the onset to the peak of the deflection wave as shown in Fig. 7.

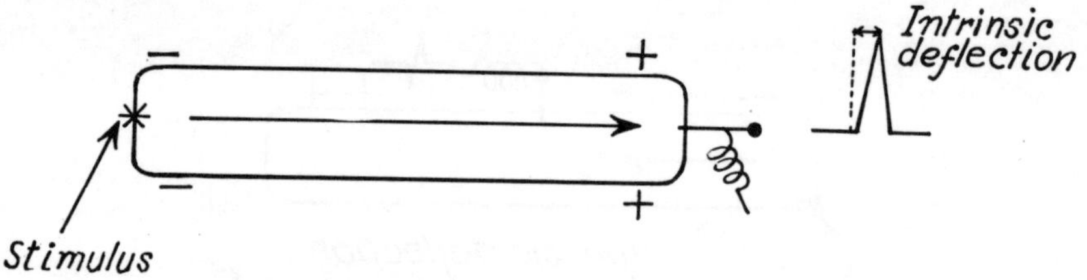

Fig. 7. A diagrammatic representation of a stimulated muscle strip showing intrinsicoid deflection time.

Repolarisation: The process of return of a stimulated muscle to its resting state is known as repolarisation.

If depolarisation occurs from the right end towards the left end of the muscle strip and the repolarisation occurs from left to right, i.e. in the opposite direction, the deflection of repolarisation i.e. of T wave, will be in the same direction as that during depolarisation. (vide fig. 8)

If depolarisation occurs from left end towards the right end of the muscle strip, and the repolarisation occurs from left to right i.e. in the same direction, the deflection of repolarisation i.e. of T wave, will be in the opposite direction to that during depolarisation as shown in fig9.

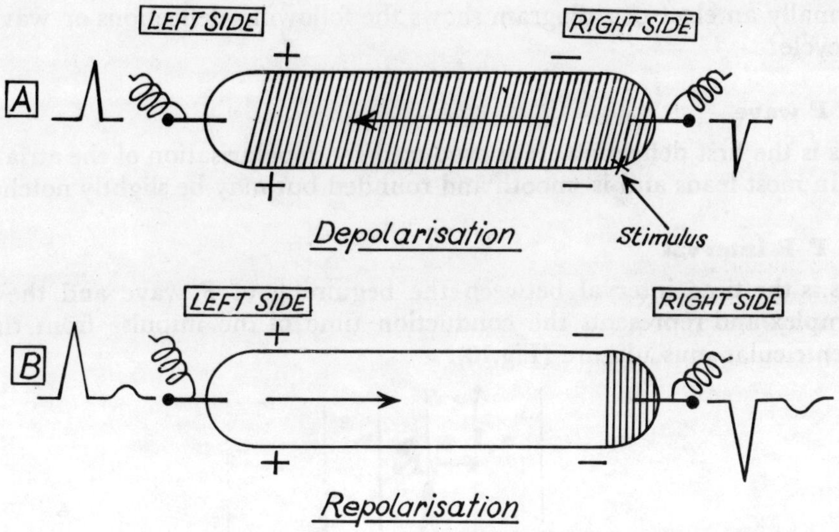

Fig. 8. A. A diagrammatic representation of a stimulated muscle strip showing depolarisation wave from right to left with deflection of the galvanometer; B. that during repolarisation from left to right.

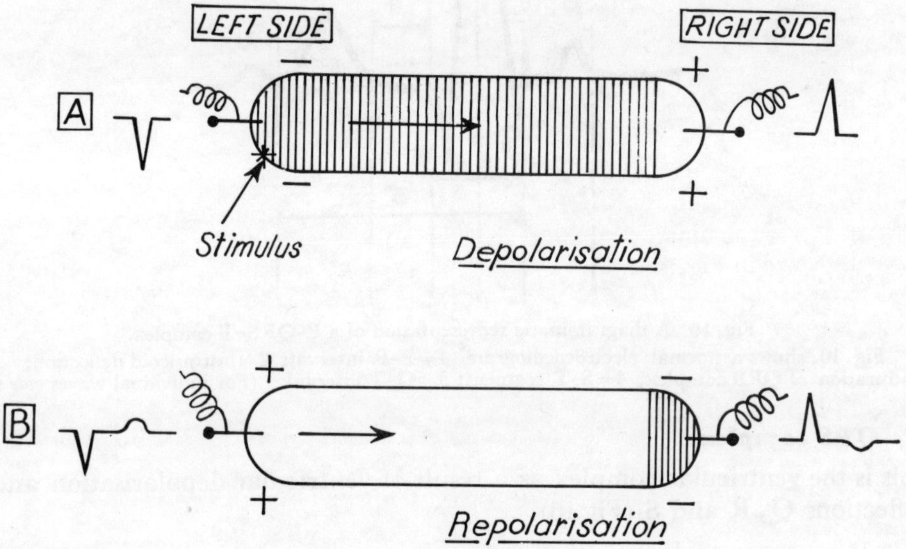

Fig. 9. A. A diagrammatic representation of a stimulated muscle strip showing depolarisation wave from left to right with deflection of the galvanometer; B. that during repolarisation from left to right.

CHAPTER III

THE NORMAL ELECTROCARDIOGRAM

Normally an electrocardiogram shows the following deflections or waves in a single cardiac cycle:

P wave

This is the first deflection. It is produced by depolarisation of the atria. It is directed upward in most leads and is smooth and rounded but may be slightly notched (Fig.10).

P–R interval

This is the time interval between the beginning of P wave and the beginning of QRS complex and represents the conduction time of the impulse from the sinus node to the ventricular musculature (Fig.10).

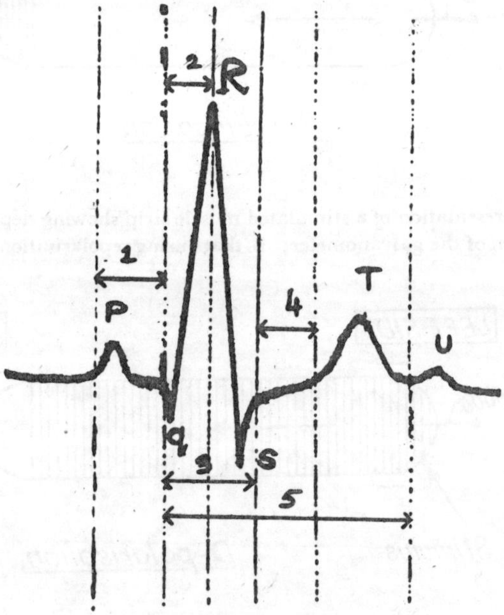

Fig. 10. A diagrammatic representation of a P–QRS–T complex.
Fig. 10. shows a normal electrocardiogram. 1=P–R interval; 2=intrinsicoid deflection; 3=duration of QRS complex; 4=S–T segment; 5=Q–T interval. (For individual waves *vide* text.)

QRS complex

This is the ventricular complex as a result of ventricular depolarisation and consists of 3 deflections Q, R and S (Fig.10).

Q wave—The first downward deflection of the QRS complex after the P wave is Q wave. It indicates depolarisation of the interventricular septum.

R wave—The first upward deflection of the QRS complex after the P wave is R wave which may or may not be preceded by a Q wave. R wave indicates ventricular depolarisation.

R′ wave—This is the second upward deflection after the R wave and may be present in conduction defects.

S wave—It is the downward deflection following R wave and indicates completion of the ventricular depolarisation.

Q–S wave—When the QRS complex consists of a downward deflection only, it is designated as a Q–S wave.

S–T segment

This is the isoelectric base line between the end of S wave and beginning of T wave **and represents the time taken for the beginning of ventricular repolarisation or recovery after its depolarisation.**

T wave

This is upward in most leads and represents ventricular repolarisation.

Q–T interval

This indicates the duration of electrical systole of the ventricles (ventricular excitation and recovery) and is measured from the beginning of the QRS complex to the end of the T wave. This varies with the heart rate and when the observed Q–T interval is corrected with the existing heart rate, it is called the corrected Q–T interval (Q–Tc); this is determined easily by using a nomogram drawn for this purpose or by using a formula (Taran and Szilagyi, 1947), viz., $Q\text{–}Tc = \frac{Q\text{–}T}{\sqrt{C}}$, Q–T being the observed Q–T interval in seconds and c representing cardiac cycle length (R–R interval) in seconds. With a heart rate of 60 per minute, the Q–Tc is 0·42 second in males and 0·43 second in females.

U wave

This small positive deflection is sometimes seen after T wave and its significance is ill-understood.

Intrinsicoid deflection (Ventricular activation time—V.A.T.)

It is the time taken by the electrical impulse to reach the ventricular surface from the left side of the interventricular septum and is measured from the beginning of Q wave or R wave (when Q wave is absent) to the peak of R wave.

The V.A.T. should not exceed 0.02 second in V_1 and 0.04 second in V_5.

NORMAL VARIATION OF ELECTROCARDIOGRAM PATTERNS IN DIFFERENT LEADS

The patterns of the different waves in the electrocardiogram are not similar in different leads; and one should be accustomed with the different normal patterns of the electrocardiogram in different leads.

P wave

The P wave is upright in leads I, II, aVF, V_4, V_5 and V_6, inverted in lead aVR and variable in leads III, aVL, V_1, V_2 and V_3 (chest leads), height and width of P wave being within normal limits.

QRS complex

The main deflection of the QRS complex may be either upward (positive) or downward (negative) or R and S waves may be equal.

In the limb leads, bipolar and unipolar, the main deflection is variable except in aVR where the main deflection is downward, i.e., a small R wave with a deep S wave, or only a Q wave (so-called Q–S wave), or a deep Q wave with a small R wave is seen (Fig.11).

In the chest leads there is a definite pattern of QRS complexes; as one goes from right ventricular surface leads towards the left ventricular surface leads, i.e., from V_1 to V_6, the initial small R wave gradually becomes taller and taller while the S wave becomes more and more diminutive in size and it may disappear completely. The lead in which the height and depth of R and S waves are almost equal is referred to as the transitional zone. Thus the patterns of QRS complexes in the V leads are as follows:

V_1 and V_2 (Right ventricular surface leads). There is a small R wave with a deep S wave in these leads (Fig.12).

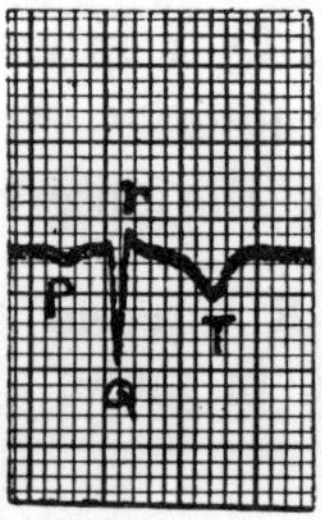

Fig. 11.

Fig. 11 shows a normal electrocardiogram from lead aVR.

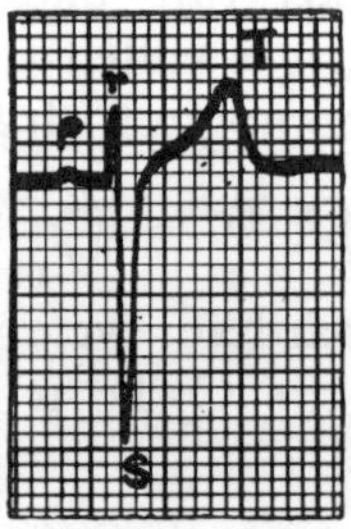

Fig. 12.

Fig. 12 is a typical electrocardiogram from lead V_1.

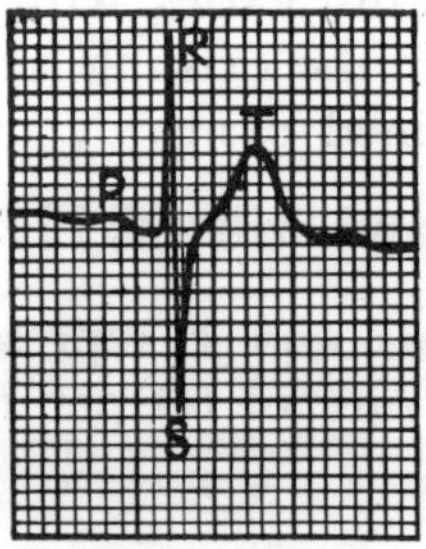

Fig. 13.

Fig. 13 shows an electrocardiogram from lead V_4.

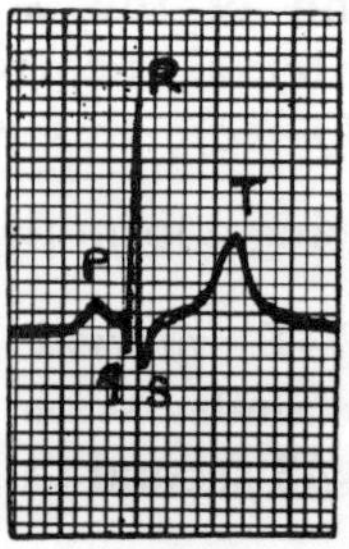

Fig. 14.

Fig. 14 is an electrocardiogram from lead V_5.

V_3 and V_4 (Transitional zone). Here the R and S waves are almost equal (Fig.13)

V_5 and V_6 (Left ventricular surface leads). Here the R wave is tall with a little or no S wave (Fig.14)

T wave

Normally the T wave is:

upright in leads I, II, aVF, V_3 to V_6,

inverted in aVR,

variable in leads III, aVL, V_1 and V_2.

PHASES OF RESPIRATION AND CHANGES IN THE PATTERNS OF ELECTROCARDIOGRAM

Sometimes when the diaphragm is high, the T wave in aVF may be flattened or inverted; in such cases aVF should be repeated in deep inspiration when the inversion of the T wave in lead aVF may be corrected and may become upright.

CHAPTER IV

METHOD OF READING AN ELECTROCARDIOGRAM

With an electrocardiogram in hand the following points are to be noted systematically for quick and correct interpretation. It may be mentioned that an electrocardiogram should always be interpreted on clinical background.

1. To note whether P wave is present in all the leads and whether each P wave is followed by a QRS complex.
2. To note whether the P–QRS–T complexes are similar in a particular lead.
3. To note whether the intervals in between the successive P–QRS–T complexes are equal.
4. To determine the heart rate—This is determined by dividing 1500 (1 minute= 1500 small squares) by the number of small squares lying between the peaks of two successive R waves, when the tracing-paper speed is 25 mm./sec. at which it is routinely kept.
5. To study the detailed patterns of individual P waves, P–R intervals, QRS complexes, S–T segments, T waves, U waves, if present, and Q–T intervals.
6. To study the electrical axis, lie, and rotation of the heart.

P wave

P wave is better seen in leads I, II, aVF and V_1. Normal duration (width) of P wave is not more than 0·1 sec. (2½ small squares) and normal height of P wave is not more than 2·5 mm.

Left atrial enlargement is recognised by a wide P wave (more than 2½ small squares), which may be notched and then the interval between two peaks of the notched P wave is more than 1 small square—**P mitrale** (Fig.15).

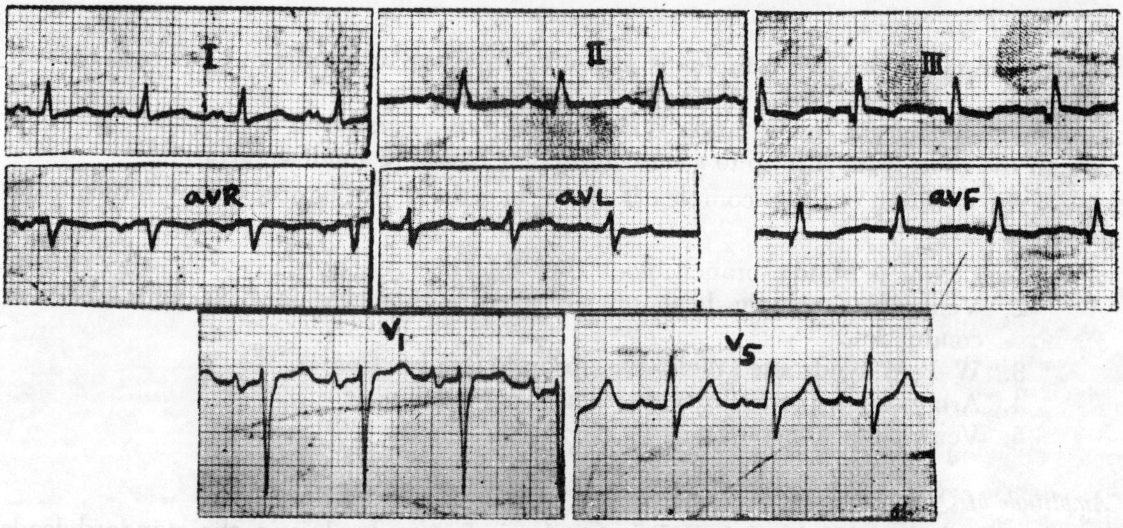

Fig.15.

Fig. 15. The electrocardiogram shows left atrial enlargement (P–mitrale) and old myocardial infarction of postero-inferior wall.

Right atrial enlargement is recognised by an increased height of P wave, i.e., more than 2½ mm. and the shape of the P wave is peaked—**P pulmonale.**

Bi-atrial enlargement is recognised by the presence of the combined features of enlargement of both the atria.

Persistent absence of P waves in all the leads may indicate atrial fibrillation and nodal rhythm. In paroxysmal ventricular tachycardia there may be a total absence or an occasional appearance of P waves.

Biphasic P wave may indicate left atrial enlargement or ectopic beat.

Inverted P waves in appropriate leads indicate nodal ectopic beats, nodal tachycardia, dextrocardia, laevocardia or ventricular tachycardia with retrograde conduction.

Garden-brick or saw-tooth appearance of P waves indicates atrial flutter.

Replacement of the P waves by fibrillary or 'f' waves indicates atrial fibrillation. 'f' waves of atrial fibrillation are best seen in lead V_1. Fibrillary waves may not be visible in any lead in some cases.

P–R interval

This should be studied in all the leads. It is measured from the beginning of P wave to the beginning of QRS complex. It should not exceed 0·22 sec. (5½ small squares).

Prolonged P–R interval, (i.e., more than 0·22 sec.) indicates 1st degree heart block.

If P–R interval is less than 0·1 sec. (2½ small squares) it may indicate atrial ectopic beat, nodal ectopic beat, and Wolff-Parkinson-White syndrome (W–P–W syndrome).

QRS complex

QRS complexes should be studied in all the leads; the pattern of the individual QRS complex in each lead should also be studied (*vide* variation in different leads).

Duration of QRS complex

The duration of QRS complex is measured from the beginning of Q wave to the end of S wave.

In the limb leads the duration is normally up to a maximum of 0·11 sec.

In the chest leads it is up to a maximum of 0·12 sec. (3 small squares).

If the duration of QRS complex is more than the above figures it may indicate the following:

1. Complete bundle-branch block (B.B.B.).
2. Ventricular ectopic beat or supraventricular ectopic beat with aberrant conduction.
3. W–P–W syndrome (Wolff-Parkinson-White syndrome).
4. Arborisation block (intraventricular conduction defect).
5. Ventricular aberration.

Amplitude of QRS complex

If the total amplitude of the QRS complex is 5 mm. or less in the standard leads (I, II, III), it is a low voltage complex. Low voltage complexes may be present in (Fig.16):

1. Diffuse coronary arterial disease.
2. Pericardial effusion, and constrictive pericarditis.
3. Myxoedema.

4. Gross cardiac failure with huge enlargement of the heart.
5. Widespread myocardial damage.

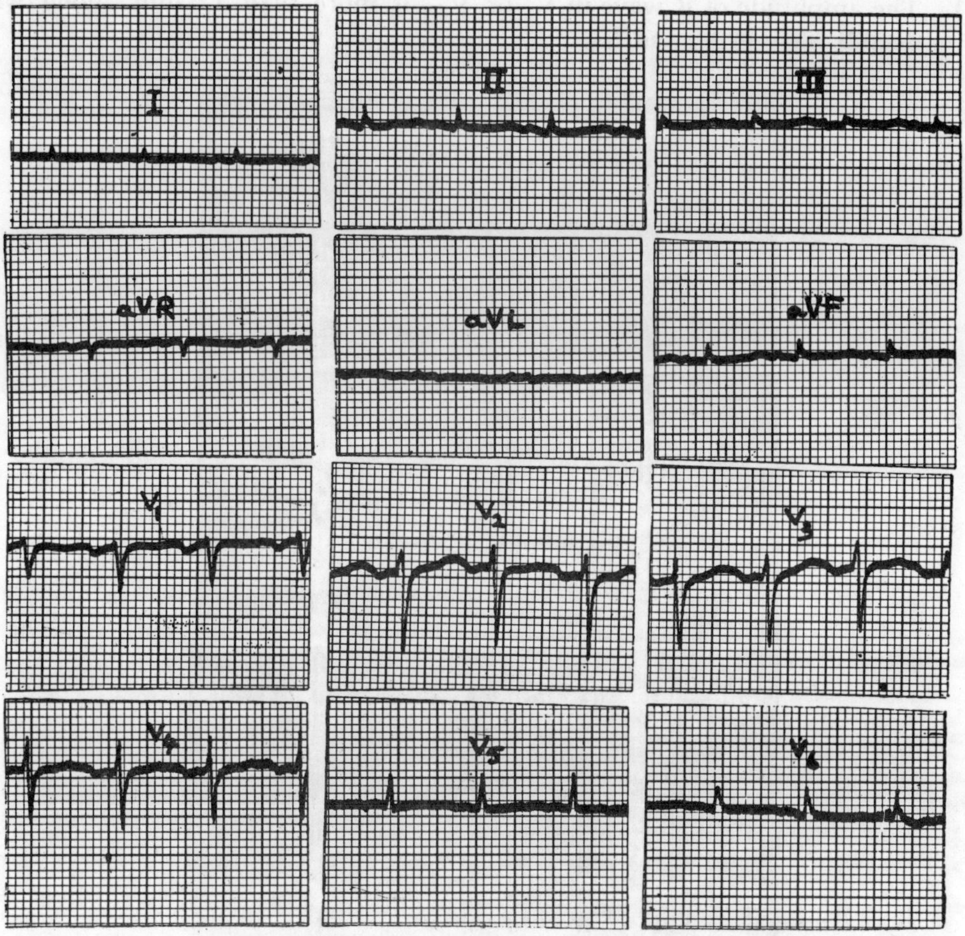

Fig. 16.

Fig. 16 shows an electrocardiogram with low voltage complexes from a case of myxoedema.

Ventricular hypertrophy patterns

Left ventricular hypertrophy is recognised when any two of the following criteria are satisfied (Fig.17):

1. The summation of the amplitude (in mm.) of R wave in V_5 and S wave in V_1 is 35 mm. or more, or that of R wave in V_6 and S wave in V_2 is 40 mm. or more.
2. R wave in V_5 or in V_6, reaches 25 mm. or more, or S wave in V_1 or V_2 reaches 25 mm. or more.
3. R or S wave in limb leads is 20 mm. or more.
4. R wave in aVF is more than 21 mm.
5. R wave in aVL is more than 13 mm.
6. QRS duration is over 0·09 sec., in standard leads or ventricular activation time is more than 0·04 sec. in V_5 and V_6.
7. Left axis deviation is $-30°$ or more.

Right ventricular hypertrophy is recognised when one of the following criteria is satisfied (Fig. 18):

1. The amplitude of R wave in V_1 or V_{3R} is more than 12 mm. along with a deep S wave in V_5 and V_6.

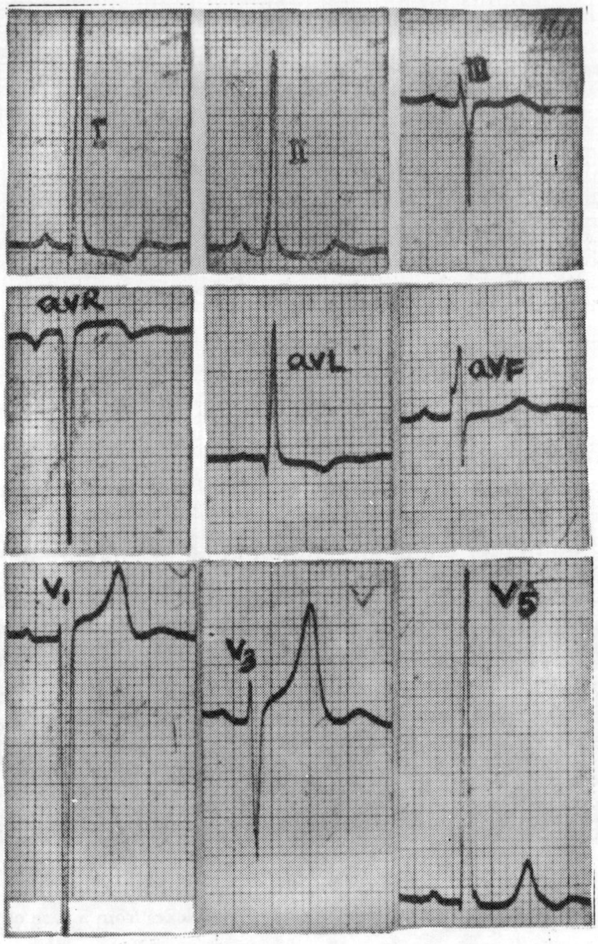

Fig. 17.

Fig. 17 shows a marked hypertrophy of the left ventricle.

2. The amplitude of R wave is 80% of or equal to or more than the depth of S wave in V_1, provided that the height of R wave is at least 7 mm. in V_1 or V_{3R}.
3. Right axis deviation is more than +110° in an adult or ventricular activation time is more than 0·02 sec. in V_1 or V_{3R}.
4. S wave is deeper than R wave in three standard leads in children.
5. An upright T wave is seen in V_1 in infant.

Systolic overloading

Systolic overloading of the left ventricle occurs in hypertension and aortic stenosis and is recognised by classical pattern of left ventricular hypertrophy such as a deep S wave over the right ventricle, a tall R wave over the left ventricle, an inversion of U wave in the left ventricular surface leads, left axis deviation, QRS duration 0·09 sec. or more, the intrinsicoid deflection in V_5 and V_6 0·04 sec. or more, depression of S–T segment with an upward convexity, and inverted T wave (Fig. 19). Left ventricular dilatation will aggravate S–T segment and T wave changes.

Systolic overloading of the right ventricle occurs in pulmonary hypertension, and pulmonary stenosis and is recognised by a marked right axis deviation, a tall R wave over the right ventricle and a deep S wave over the left ventricle with depression of S–T segment and inversion of T wave in V_1, V_2, V_3 and V_{3R}.

Diastolic overloading

Diastolic overloading of the left ventricle occurs in aortic and mitral incompetence, patent ductus arteriosus, etc., and is recognised by a prominent, upright and pointed T wave in V_5 and V_6 along with a tall R wave over the left ventricle and a deep S wave over the right ventricle (Fig. 20). P wave may show P–mitrale pattern.

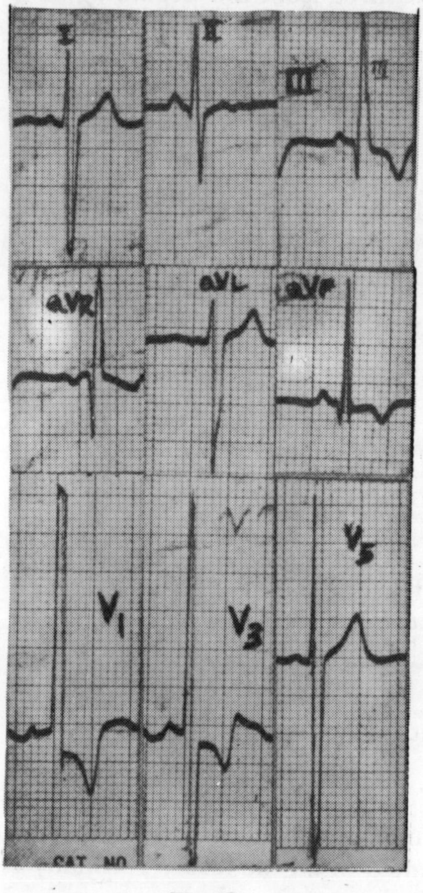

Fig. 18.
Fig. 18 shows a marked hypertrophy of the right ventricle with strain.

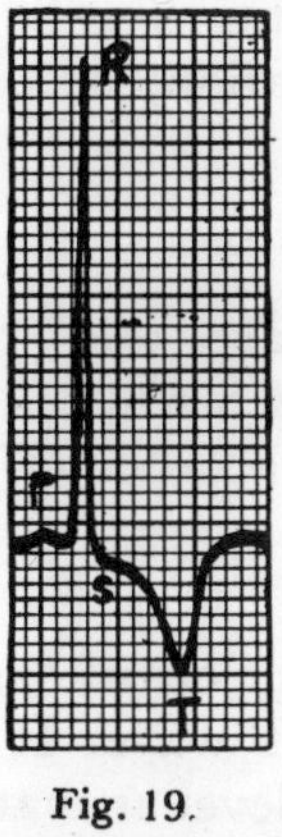

Fig. 19.
Fig. 19 shows a tracing from lead V_5 in systolic overloading of left ventricle.

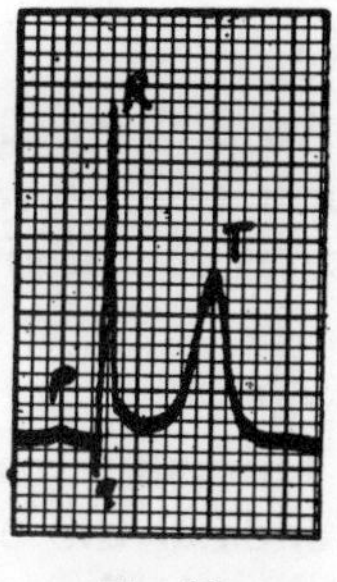

Fig. 20.
Fig. 20 shows a tracing from lead V_5 in diastolic overloading of left ventricle.

Diastolic overloading of the right ventricle occurs in atrial septal defect and is recognised by the presence of a complete or incomplete right bundle-branch block pattern in the electrocardiogram usually indicating hypertrophy of the basal portion of the right ventricle.

Strain pattern

This term is used when the S–T segment is depressed with an upward convexity and blends with the proximal limb of the asymmetrically inverted T wave. The condition develops when there is ventricular hypertrophy followed by ventricular dilatation and failure probably as a result of myocardial ischaemia and conduction defects. In acute ventricular strain there may be a bundle-branch block. Ventricular strain may be an indirect evidence of ventricular hypertrophy.

Individual waves of QRS complex

Q wave

A careful search should always be made for the presence of Q waves in ventricular complexes. Normally its duration (width) is less than 0·04 sec. (i.e., less than one small square) and its depth is not more than 2 mm. and is measured from the beginning of Q wave to the beginning of R wave.

A large Q wave in appropriate leads may indicate myocardial infarction or necrosis, or ventricular aneurysm.

R wave

A normal R wave is usually sharply pointed. If R wave is notched or slurred it usually indicates conduction defect in absence of technical fault in the tracing (Fig. 21).

Intrinsicoid deflection

This is to be examined in leads V_1 and V_5 or V_6. In V_1 it is up to 0·02 sec. (i.e., $\frac{1}{2}$ small square) normally. In V_5 or V_6 it is up to 0·04 sec. (i.e., one small square) normally. Increased intrinsicoid deflection indicates ventricular hypertrophy or dilatation, or conduction defect.

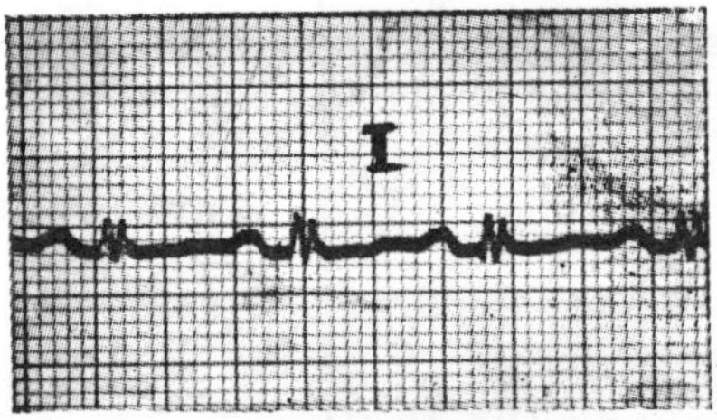

Fig. 21.

Fig. 21 shows a tracing in lead I from a case of left bundle-branch block (M–shaped complex).

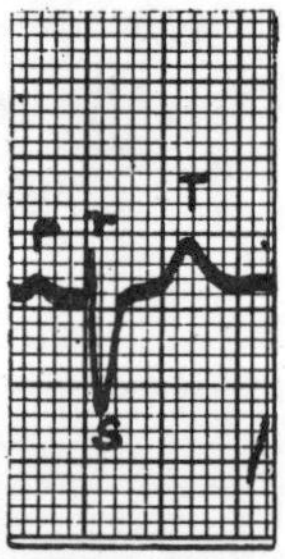

Fig. 22.

Fig. 22 shows a slurred S wave.

S wave

An S wave should be sharp and uniform as R wave. Slurring of S wave indicates conduction defect in absence of technical fault in the tracing (Fig. 22).

S–T segment

This is the part of the electrocardiogram which immediately follows QRS complex, and ends at the beginning of T wave. It should be studied in all the leads. Normally it is isoelectric (i.e., at the same level as that of the base line).

An elevation of S–T segment up to 1 mm. in the limb leads and up to 2 mm. in the chest leads is normal.

A depression of S–T segment up to 0·5 mm. (i.e., $\frac{1}{2}$ small square) may be normal.

An abnormal elevation of the S–T segment indicates acute myocardial infarction, or pericarditis, or ventricular aneurysm.

An abnormal depression of S–T segment indicates myocardial ischaemia, digitalis effect, or subendocardial infarction.

Normally S–T segment is not an absolutely straight horizontal line. If it is so, for more than a length of 2 small squares, it is suspicious of myocardial ischaemia (Fig. 23).

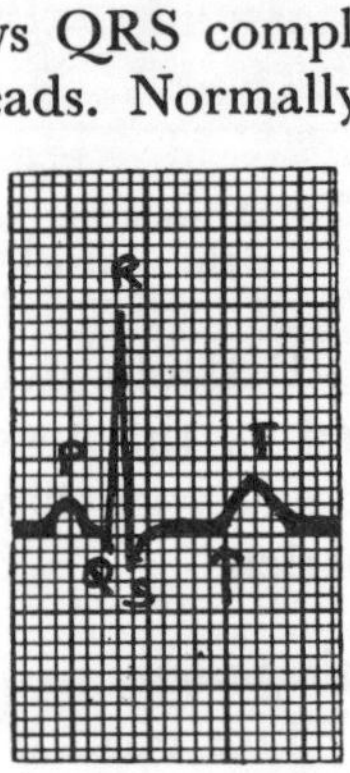

Fig. 23.

Fig. 23 shows an absolutely horizontal S–T segment for more than 2 small squares which is suspicious of myocardial ischaemia.

In some cases there may be sagging of S–T segment which

is also abnormal and may occur after digitalis administration, in hypokalaemia, and in ventricular strain.

T wave

T wave follows the S–T segment and it should be studied in all the leads. Normally it is upright in leads I, II, aVF, V_3, V_4, V_5 and V_6; it is inverted in aVR and variable in leads III, aVL, V_1 and V_2.

Abnormality in T wave may be seen as a low, flattened, biphasic or an inverted T wave. An abnormal T wave may indicate:

1. Myocardial infarction.
2. Coronary insufficiency.
3. Ventricular strain.
4. Non-specific myocardial changes.
5. Digitalis effect.
6. Myxoedema.
7. Hypokalaemia.

The pattern where the two limbs of the inverted T wave are similar in slope and length (symmetrically inverted T wave), indicates myocardial infarction.

Pointed, upright, tall T waves usually indicate hyperkalaemia, and sometimes ischaemic heart disease.

Q–T interval

The corrected Q–T interval may be determined from the R–R interval and observed Q–T interval of the tracing from a recognised monogram. Q–Tc interval may be prolonged in myocarditis, hypokalcaemia and hypothermia at 30°C. and shortened in hyperkalcaemia and after digitalisation.

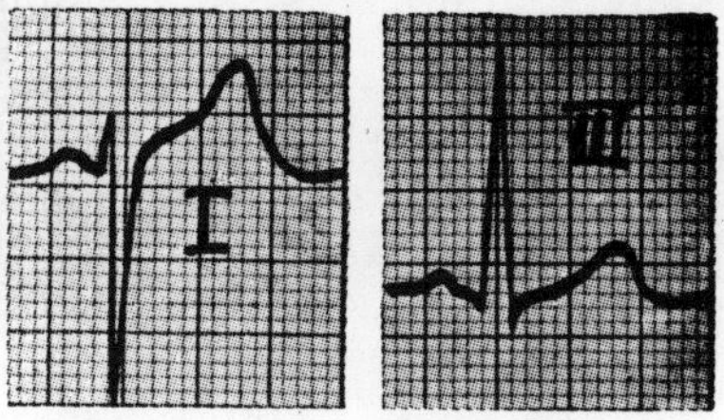

Fig. 24.
Fig. 24 shows a right axis deviation.

U wave

A prominent U wave occurs in hypokalaemia.

An inverted U wave may indicate ventricular strain.

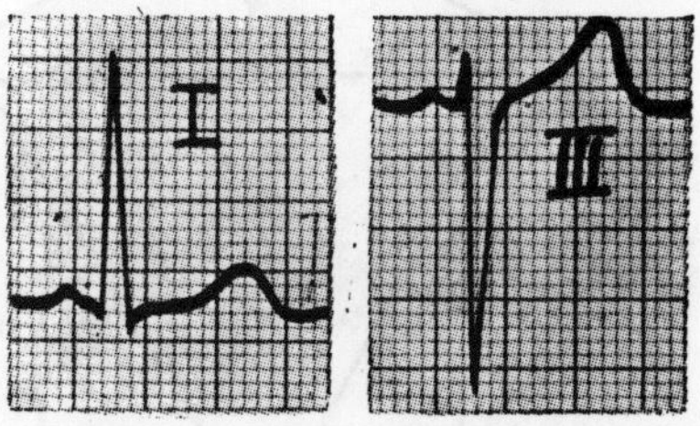

Fig. 25.
Fig. 25 shows a left axis deviation.

Determination of the axis

The electrical axis of the heart may be normal, or it may be deviated to the right or left (Figs. 24 & 25).

Leads I and III are to be examined to determine the axis. If there is no large S wave compared to the R wave in these leads, the axis is normal.

If lead I shows a deeper S wave than the height of R wave and lead III shows a taller R wave than the depth of S wave, the axis is right.

If lead III shows a deeper S wave than the height of R wave and lead I shows a taller R wave than the depth of S wave, the axis is left.

Right axis usually occurs in right ventricular hypertrophy and left axis in left ventricular hypertrophy.

THE TRI-AXIAL REFERENCE SYSTEM

The electrical axis of the heart may also be expressed in degrees, and determined by using the tri-axial reference system which is obtained as follows: the three sides AB, AC and BC of an Einthoven Triangle ABC (Fig. 26) representing the three bipolar standard leads I, II and III respectively are made to intersect each other at their midpoint 'O' which represents the centre of the electrical activity of the heart; thus the three hundred and sixty degrees are divided into six equal segments by these three straight lines.

Conventionally the pole 'B' (the positive pole of lead I) is taken to be 0°, the other pole 'A' as ±180°; the poles above the line AB are negative, and those below are positive (Fig. 26).

Now each of these straight lines is divided into small equal segments.

To determine the electrical axis of the heart, the algebraic sum of the R and S waves of QRS complexes in any two standard leads in mm. is plotted in the negative or the

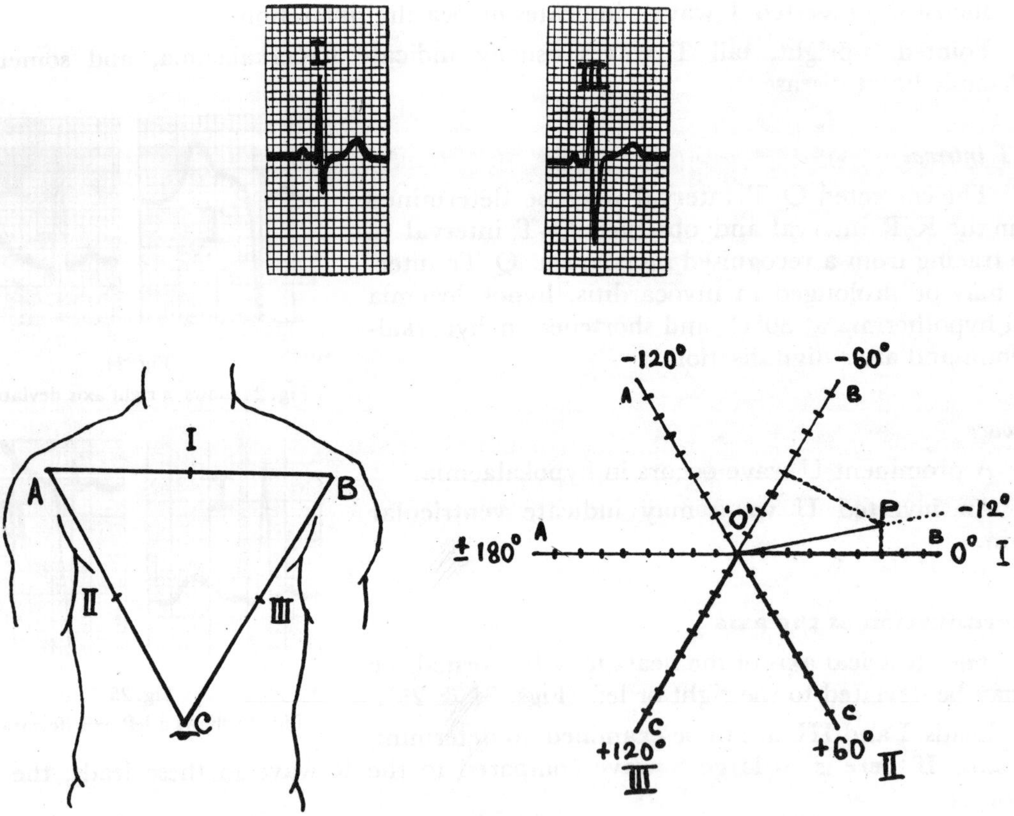

Fig. 26.
Fig. 26 shows the method of determining the electrical axis of the heart from the tri-axial reference system (*vide* text).

positive side of the respective lead axes of the tri-axial reference system (Fig. 26). In the illustration given here the algebraic sum of the R and S waves in lead I is +6 mm. and that in lead III is −4 mm. So the value +6 is plotted in the positive side (thick line) of the lead I axis at a distance of 6 segments from the centre 'O'; similarly the value −4 is plotted in the negative side (thin line) of the lead III axis at a distance of 4 segments from the centre. A perpendicular is dropped from each of these points to intersect each other at a point P. The points P and 'O' are now joined by a straight line, and thus the angle POB in degrees is the electrical axis of the given electrocardiogram, which is −12° in this case.

If the electrical axis of the heart, thus obtained, lies between 0° and +90° it is normal, if it is 0° to −90° it is left axis, and if it is +90° to ±180° it is right axis. So the illustrated case has left axis deviation.

The recent and widely accepted criteria to differentiate the abnormal axis deviations from the normal right and left axis deviations are as follows: the axis between −30° and +110° is normal, the axis between −30° and −90° is abnormal left axis deviation, and the axis between +110° and ±180° is abnormal right axis deviation.

Determination of the lie

The lie may be horizontal, vertical or intermediate. Leads aVL and aVF help in determining the lie (Figs. 27 & 28).

If there is no deep S wave in these leads, the lie is intermediate.

If there is a deeper S wave in aVL with a taller R wave in aVF compared to R wave and S wave in the respective leads, the lie is vertical.

If there is a deeper S wave in aVF with a taller R wave in aVL compared to R wave and S wave in the respective leads, the lie is horizontal.

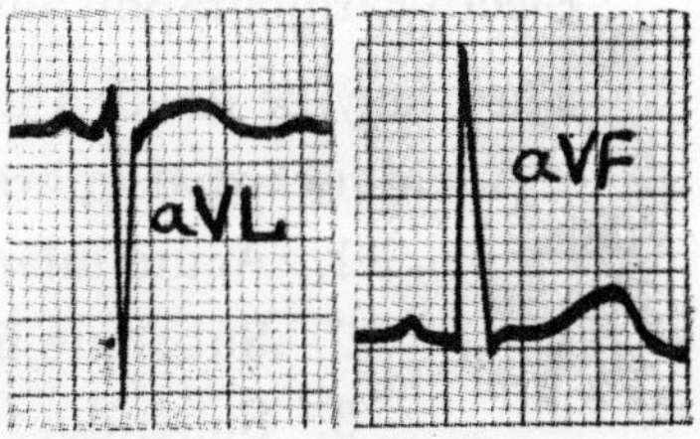

Fig. 27.

Fig. 27 shows a tracing from leads aVL and aVF indicating a vertical lie.

Determination of the rotation

Electrically the heart may be rotated in a clockwise or anticlockwise direction.

In the chest leads the position of the transitional zone, i.e., the lead in which almost equal height and depth of R and S waves are found, is to be examined for determining the rotation. If the transitional zone is situated in V_3 and V_4, i.e., QRS complex shows equal height and depth of R and S waves in these leads, there is no rotation of the heart.

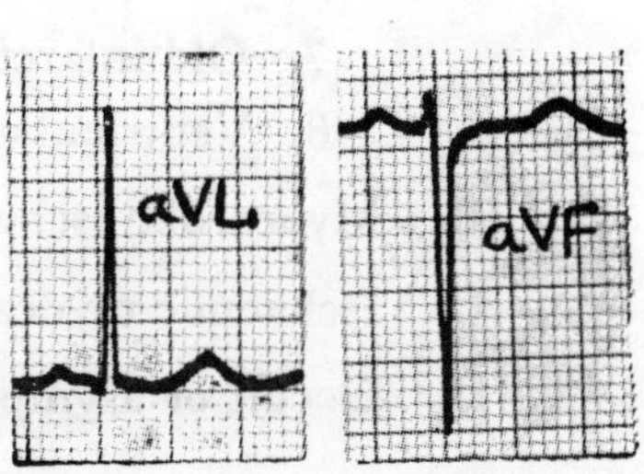

Fig. 28.

Fig. 28 shows a tracing from leads aVL and aVF indicating a horizontal lie.

If the transitional zone is shifted to the left ventricular surface leads (V_5 and V_6) or if there is a big S wave in these leads, the rotation is clockwise.

If the transitional zone is shifted to the right ventricular surface leads (V_1 and V_2) with absence of S wave in V_5 and V_6, the rotation is anticlockwise.

CHAPTER V

ISCHAEMIC HEART DISEASE

Interpretation of an electrocardiogram on clinical background is essential for the diagnosis of ischaemic heart disease (I.H.D.). Before diagnosing ischaemic heart disease in electrocardiogram one should be definite that the patient is not getting digitalis for at least 3 weeks prior to the recording of an electrocardiogram. The patient should be in empty stomach before the recording is done.

Ventricular walls involved in I.H.D. may be recognised by studying the leads indicated below:

1. Anterior wall ... Lead I with or without II.
2. Postero-inferior wall ... Leads III, aVF with or without II.
3. Septal wall ... Leads V_3 and V_4.
4. Lateral wall ... Leads V_5 and V_6.
5. Antero-septal wall ... Leads I, V_3, V_4 with or without II.
6. Antero-lateral wall ... Leads I, V_5, V_6 with or without II.
7. Postero-lateral wall ... Leads II, III, aVF and V_6.

Electrocardiographically ischaemic heart diseases are encountered in various forms. They may be divided into the following groups:

A. Myocardial infarction:
   1. Acute infarction.
   2. Subacute infarction.
   3. Subendocardial infarction.
   4. Subepicardial infarction.
   5. Intramural infarction.
   6. Myocardial infarction with unusual electrocardiographic findings.
   7. Old infarction.
   8. Ventricular aneurysm.

B. Myocardial ischaemia.

C. Ischaemic myocardial changes.

D. Occult or asymptomatic coronary artery disease.

A. Myocardial infarction

1. The electrocardiographic changes in **acute myocardial infarction** may conveniently be classified in the following headings:

(*a*) Acute myocardial infarction (*vide* Figs. 33–36).
(*b*) Recent myocardial infarction (*vide* Figs. 36 and 37).
(*c*) Myocardial infarction of some duration (*vide* Fig. 38).

Acute myocardial infarction

This is indicated by S–T segment elevation. This elevated S–T segment shows an upward convexity (coving). Associated with an elevated S–T segment there is usually a deep and wide (0·04 sec. or more) Q wave (Fig. 29). T wave is usually absorbed in the elevated S–T segment.

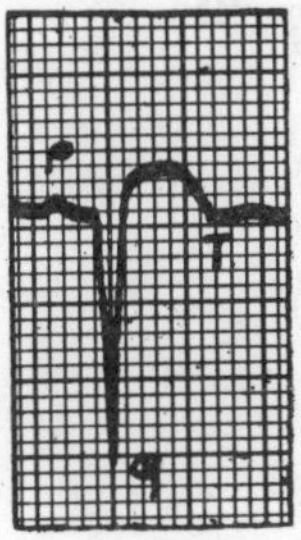

Fig. 29.

Fig. 29 shows a typical tracing which is seen in a case of acute myocardial infarction.

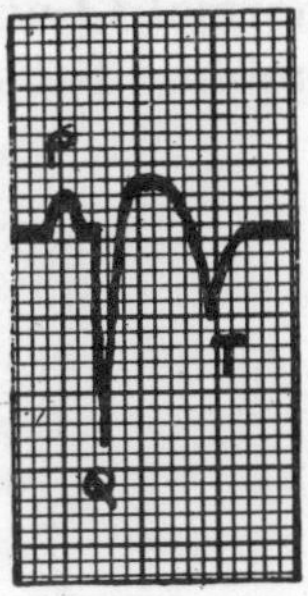

Fig. 30.

Fig. 30 shows a typical electrocardiogram which is seen in a case of recent myocardial infarction.

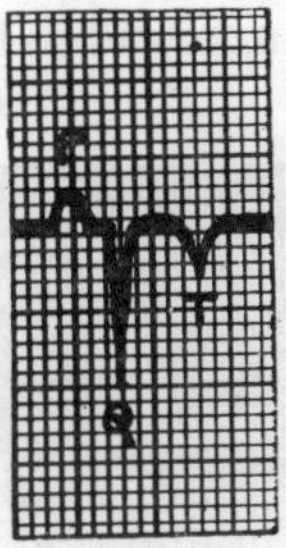

Fig. 31.

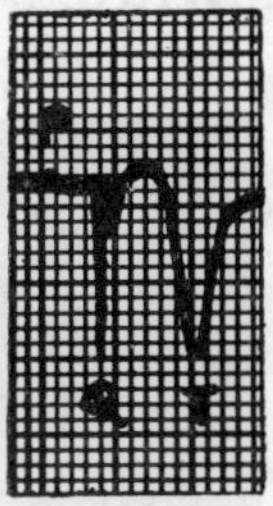

Fig. 32.

Figs. 31 and 32 show typical electrocardiograms which are found in myocardial infarction of some duration.

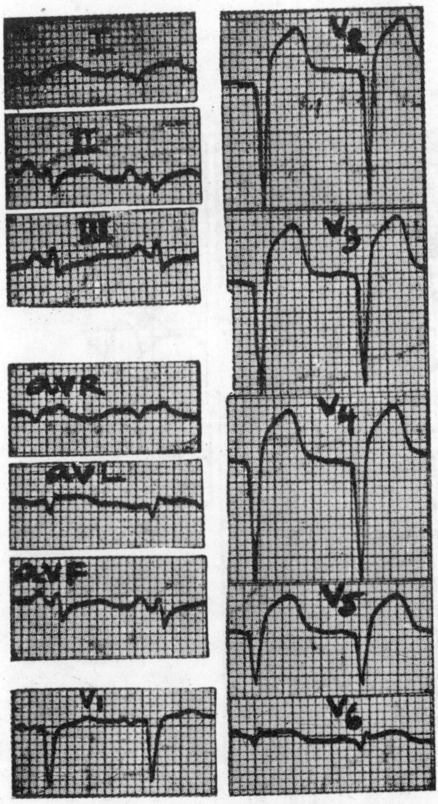

Fig. 33.

Fig. 33 shows an electrocardiogram from a case of acute myocardial infarction of antero-septal and lateral wall taken 24 hours after the clinical attack.

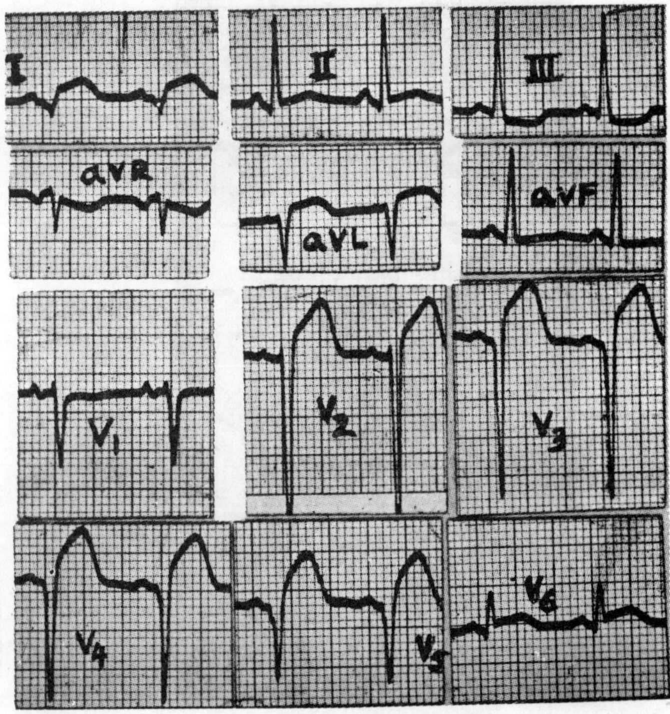

Fig. 34.

Fig. 34 shows an electrocardiogram from a case of acute myocardial infarction of antero-septal and lateral wall taken 30 hours after the clinical attack.

Recent myocardial infarction

This is indicated by the presence of an abnormal Q wave, slight elevation of S–T segment with coving, and inverted T wave which usually shows asymmetrical limbs (Fig. **30**).

Myocardial infarction of some duration

This is indicated by the presence of an abnormal Q wave, isoelectric S–T segment with inverted, pointed, symmetrical T wave resembling Bat's wing (Fig. **31**).

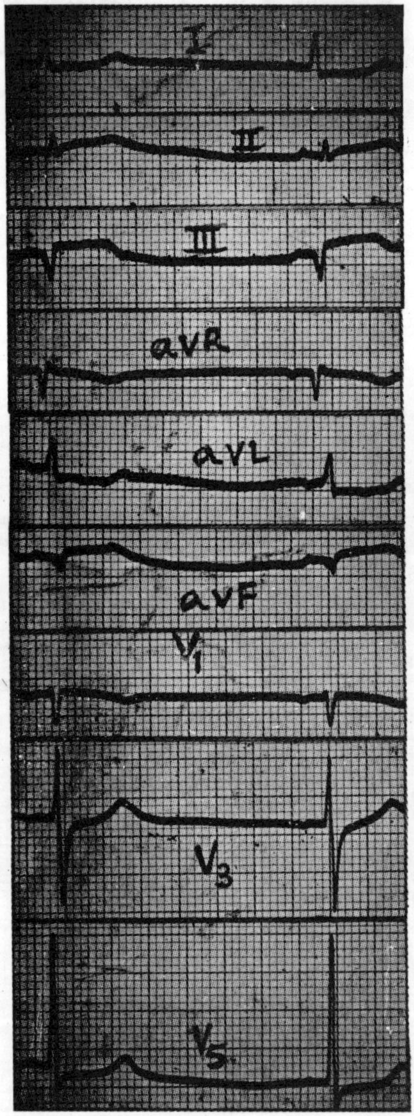

Fig. 35.

Fig. 35 shows an electrocardiogram from a case of acute myocardial infarction of postero-inferior wall taken 12 hours after the clinical attack. There is also sinus bradycardia.

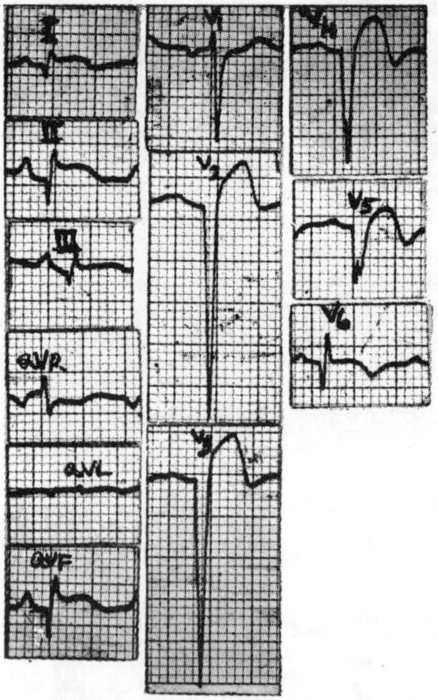

Fig. 36.

Fig. 36 shows an electrocardiogram from a case of acute myocardial infarction of postero-inferior wall and recent myocardial infarction of antero-septal and lateral wall taken 6 days after the clinical attack.

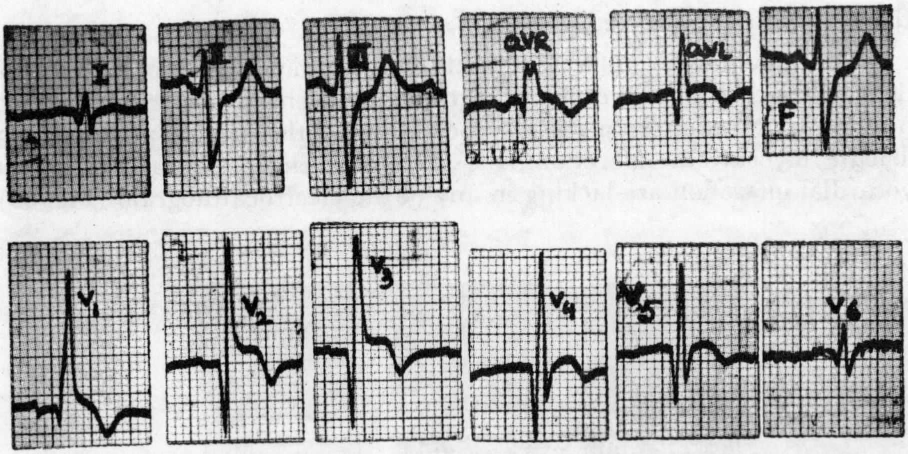

Fig. 37.

Fig. 37 shows a tracing from a case of recent myocardial infarction of antero-septal and lateral wall with a right bundle-branch block taken 5 days after the clinical attack.

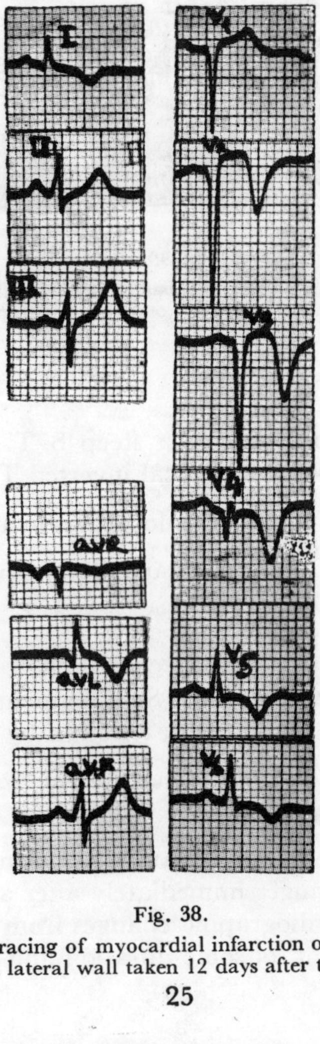

Fig. 38.

Fig. 38 shows a tracing of myocardial infarction of some duration of antero-septal and lateral wall taken 12 days after the clinical attack.

2. **Subacute myocardial infarction**

In a case of myocardial infarction if the appearance of the electrocardiographic changes is similar to that of the electrocardiographic changes of recent infarction or infarction of some duration from the very beginning of the clinical attack, it is referred to as subacute myocardial infarction. In such cases electrocardiographic features of acute myocardial infarction are lacking in any of the electrocardiogram (Fig. 39)

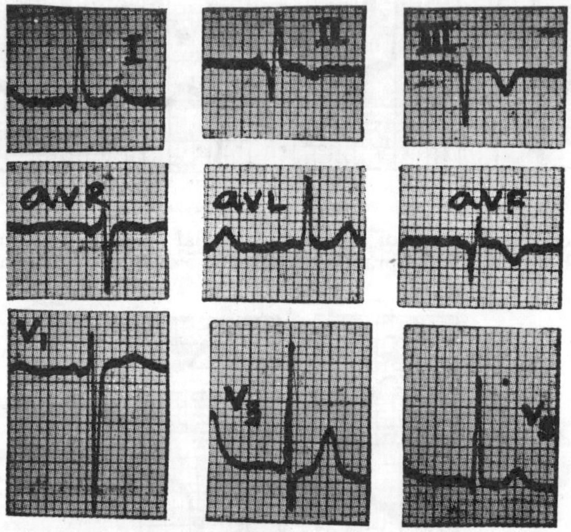

Fig. 39.

Fig. 39 shows a tracing of subacute myocardial infarction taken half an hour after the onset of the precordial pain.

3. **Subendocardial infarction**

This is diagnosed by the presence of a steep S–T segment depression (3 mm. or more), and deep, pointed, usually symmetrical inverted T waves in appropriate leads.

There is no abnormal Q wave in subendocardial infarction (Figs. 40 & 41).

Sometimes the term Acute Coronary Insufficiency is used in such cases.

4. **Subepicardial infarction**

This is indicated by an elevation of the S–T segment with coving, but without any Q wave. This is accompanied by, or later on, followed by T wave changes (Fig. 42).

5. **Intramural myocardial infarction**

This is diagnosed when there is a significant Q wave in the electrocardiogram without any S–T segment or T wave changes immediately after an acute attack of cardiac pain thus distinguishing the electrocardiographic changes from that of transmural myocardial infarctions (acute, subacute, recent, of some duration and old).

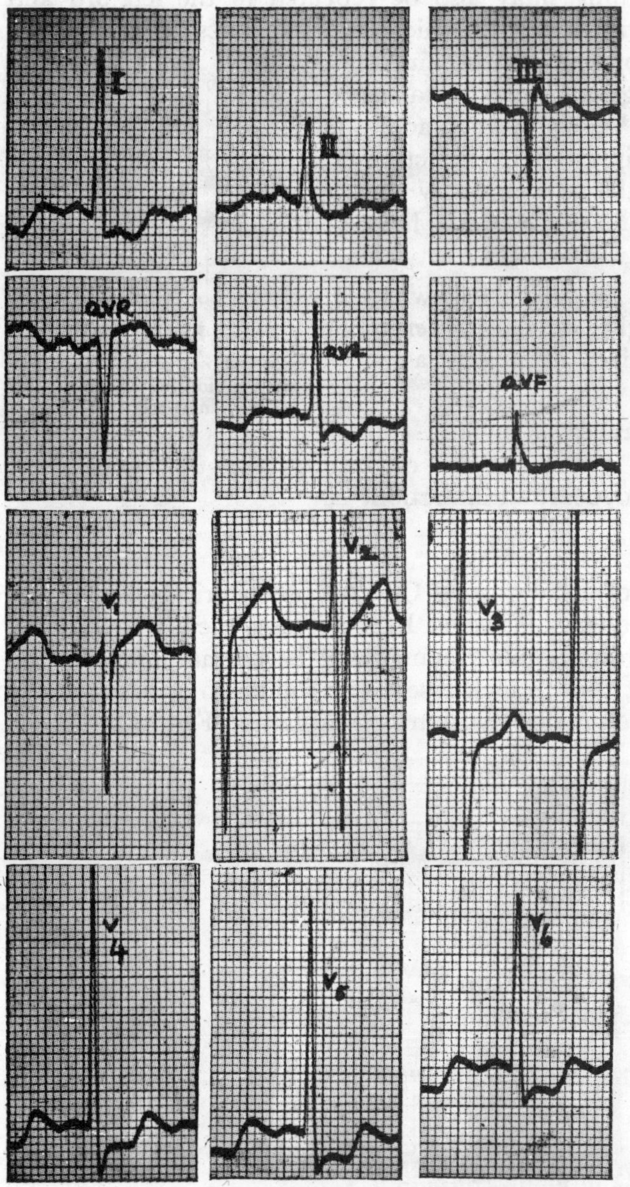

Fig. 40.

Fig. 40 shows a tracing of subendocardial infarction of antero-septal and lateral wall. There is also left ventricular hypertrophy.

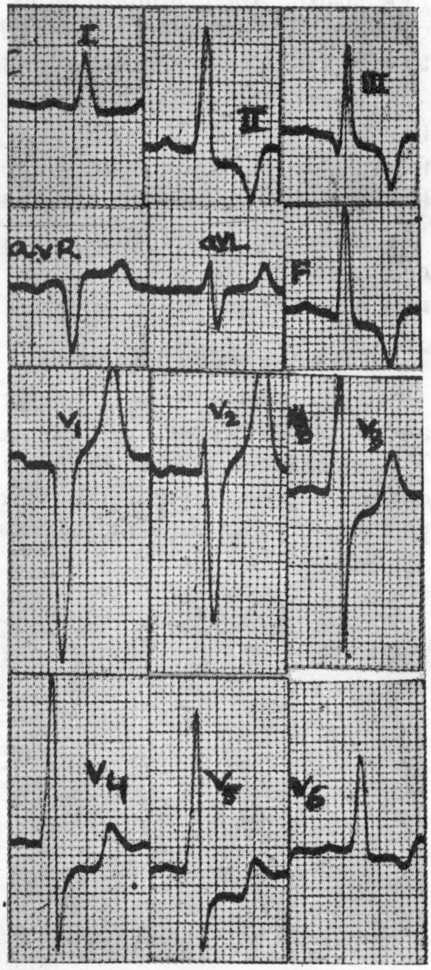

Fig. 41.

Fig. 41 shows an electrocardiogram of subendocardial infarction of antero-septal and lateral wall with left ventricular hypertrophy and left bundle-branch block.

6. Myocardial infarction with unusual electrocardiographic findings

In some rare patients with a history suggestive of acute myocardial infarction, the electrocardiogram may look apparently normal, specially if it is taken within a few hours of the clinical attack. The electrocardiogram may reveal characteristic finding if it is taken later and repeated to note gradual changes in the pattern of the tracing. The electrocardiogram showing negative findings may also be repeated in the left 3rd and 4th intercostal spaces in the left parasternal and mid-clavicular lines when characteristic findings of myocardial infarction may be obtained. In some rare instances electrocardiograms may be taken in unipolar chest leads V_7, V_8, and V_9 or after placing the exploring electrode over the xiphisternal junction (V_E lead), when abnormalities in the tracing may be obtained. Unipolar oesophageal lead may sometimes help to detect occult myocardial infarction.

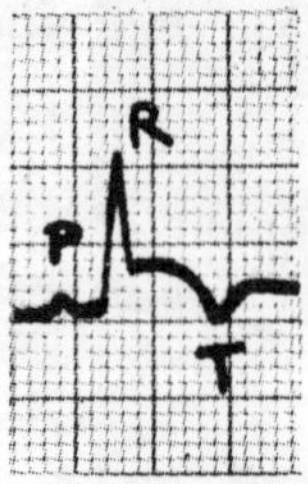

Fig. 42.

Fig. 42 shows a diagrammatic representation of subepicardial infarction.

Myocardial infarction may also be suspected when the R wave of V leads loses height as one observes from V_1 to V_6 leads, instead of gaining in height as is found in a normal electrocardiogram.

However, in all these circumstances, a white cell count, erythrocyte sedimentation rate, serum enzyme estimations and X-ray of chest may help to confirm the diagnosis of myocardial infarction.

7. Old myocardial infarction

This is indicated by the presence of an abnormal Q wave, isoelectric S–T segment and normal or biphasic or flattened or inverted T wave. In some cases there may be only T wave changes. Rarely the electrocardiographic tracing may be normal following the changes of acute myocardial infarction; thus in such cases there will be no evidence of the past infarction in the later tracings which may be within normal limits (Fig. 43).

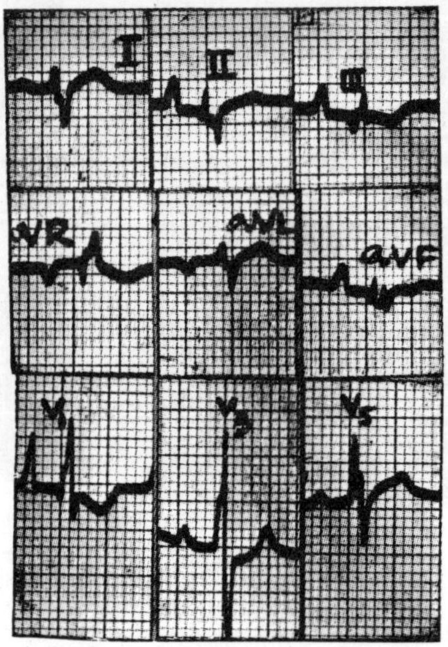

Fig. 43.

Fig. 43 shows an electrocardiogram from a case of old myocardial infarction of postero-inferior wall having congestive cardiac failure, taken 48 days after the onset of the clinical attack. There is also right atrial enlargement and right ventricular dominance.

8. **Ventricular aneurysm**

After an attack of acute myocardial infarction changes in the electrocardiogram tracing such as a prominent Q wave, elevated S–T segment and T wave inversion may persist for months or even years (Fig. 44). Under such circumstances the affected ventricular wall has developed aneurysm which may be demonstrated by further investigations such as fluoroscopy, X-ray of heart, angiocardiography and kymography.

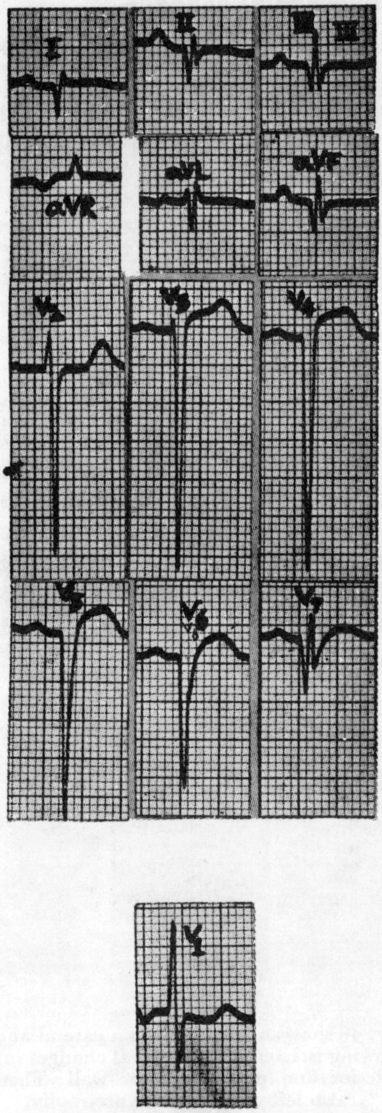

Fig. 44.

Fig. 44 shows a tracing from a case of ventricular aneurysm taken 10 months after the onset of acute myocardial infarction (proved by fluoroscopy and angiocardiography).

B. Myocardial ischaemia

Depression of S–T segment to more than ½ mm. with or without T wave changes in any lead, indicates myocardial ischaemia. When the S–T segment is slopping, the proximal part of the S–T segment should be horizontal at least for 0·08 sec. (2 small squares) to suggest myocardial ischaemia (Fig. 45).

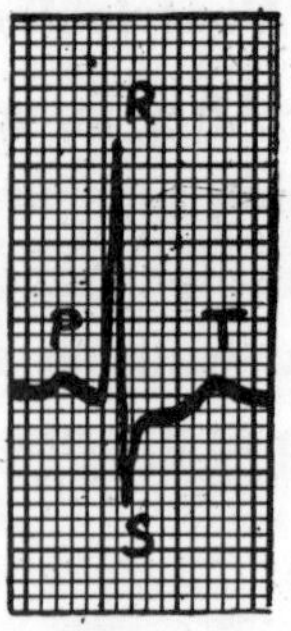

Fig. 45.
Fig. 45 is a diagrammatic representation of myocardial ischaemia.

C. Ischaemic myocardial changes

When there is a depression of the S–T segment along with T wave changes (flattening or biphasic or inversion of the T wave) the term Ischaemic Myocardial Changes is used (Fig. 46). But only T wave changes may also be due to non-specific myocardial changes.

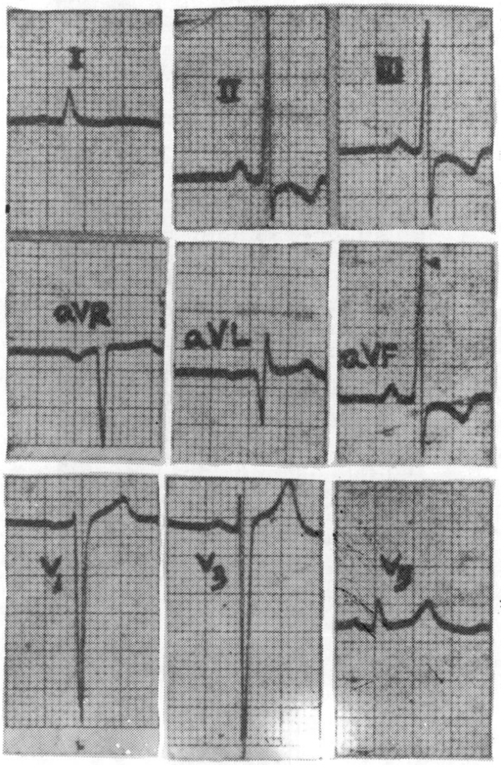

Fig. 46.
Fig. 46 shows a tracing from a case of angina showing ischaemic myocardial changes in the anterior and postero-inferior wall. There is also left ventricular hypertrophy.

D. Occult or Asymptomatic coronary artery disease

Some subjects do not have any symptom of heart disease, although electrocardiograms of these subjects show different patterns of abnormality.

On the other hand some persons may have praecordial pain of cardiac origin but their electrocardiograms taken at rest do not show any type of definite abnormality. The value of resting electrocardiogram is very little in such cases. Other methods of taking electrocardiograms have been devised in such cases.

Persons who are engaged in responsible jobs such as air-line pilots, bus drivers, etc., may require checking of their electrocardiograms to exclude coronary artery disease which may be present without any symptom. The electrocardiograms of such persons may show arrhythmias, conduction defects, evidences of myocardial infarction, S—T segment depression and T wave changes (Fig. 47). Detection of occult coronary artery disease may be further helped by post-exercise electrocardiogram, exercising electrocardiogram (i.e., electrocardiogram taken during the exercise) and coronary arteriography.

Electrocardiographic tracing during and after exercise

Sometimes the electrocardiogram may be absolutely normal in a case of angina pectoris or effort angina; in such cases if the electrocardiogram is taken immediately after exercise it may show abnormal depression of S—T segment indicating myocardial ischaemia; exercise that may be given to the patient consists of standing erect from squatting position 20 times or stepping in and out of the Master's Steps 20 times or hopping 20 times or sitting up from the recumbent posture in bed 20 times. If in the middle of the exercise the patient feels anginal pain, or is unusually breathless then the exercise should be stopped and the electrocardiogram is taken immediately (Fig. 47).

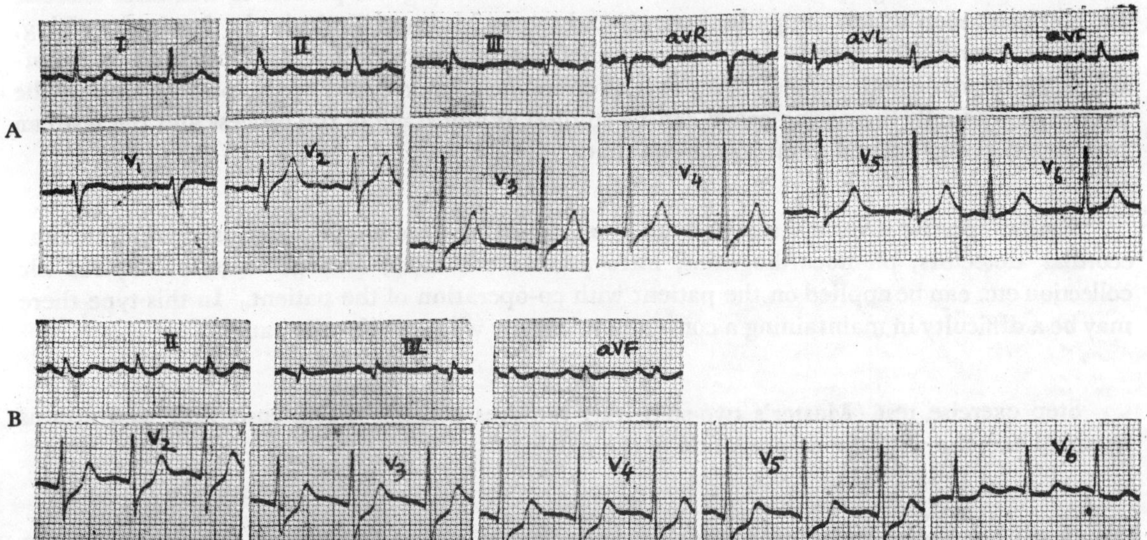

Fig. 47.

Fig. 47-A shows a tracing from a case of effort angina indicating no abnormality.

Fig 47-B shows the same tracing after exercise having depression of S-T segment indicating myocardial ischaemia.

Sometimes S–T segment depression in a case of anginal pain may revert to normal by the time the electrocardiogram is taken after the exercise. Under such circumstances, the electrocardiogram may be taken during the exercise by operating the electrocardiograph by means of radio-waves; this is called radio-electrocardiography. Exercising electrocardiogram may also be taken by using a treadmill or bicycle ergometer (Fig. 48 & 49)

With regard to exercise testing there are two types of exercises, namely, static exercise and dynamic exercise. Although static exercise or isometric exercise received considerable attention on patients of coronary arterial disease because of its popularity, this is nothing like a high-performance dynamic exercise test. After a moderate isometric exercise such as a firm, sustained hand-grip, there is a rise of systemic vascular resistance causing about a one-third increase of mean arterial pressure and about 20%. increase in heart rate. The static exercise test is only helpful in a patient having a low anginal thereshold. This type of exercise test causes an increase in cardiac work which may provoke clinical angina pectoris or ventricular dysfunction.

Dynamic exercise test involves measurement of maximal exercise capacity such as that measured by *motor-driven treadmill test* or *by upright bicycle ergometer test.*

The treadmill provides exercise suitable for both sedentary and active persons who can attain their maximal oxygen consumption. The treadmill requires a space, is noisy and expensive, and is not suitable for a patient with an indwelling vascular catheter or a sensitive praecordial detector such as a echocardiograph or a scintillation camera. During the process of treadmill exercise the platform upon which the patient stands and moves his lower limbs in the form of walking, moves at a controlled speed, and electrocardiographic, heart rate and blood pressure recordings can be made and studied. Any sort of discomfort experienced by the patient during the process of gradually increasing speed can be studied at any stage of the process and the test can be stopped at any desired point by the examiner.

Similar exercise stress test can be done by *an upright bicycle ergometer.* In this test sensible praecordial detectors, phonocardiograms, intravascular catheters, arrangements for expired air collection etc. can be applied on the patient with co-operation of the patient. In this type there may be a difficulty in maintaining a constant and steady work rate by the patient.

Step exercise test (Master's two-step test) requires a small space, costs little and attains maximal exercise with the co-operation of the patient.

In all the above tests it is convenient to undertake subjective maximal exercise test where the subject does exercises in a standard work pattern till intolerable fatigue, dyspnoea or pain supervenes.

After the graded exercise test the target heart rate at about 45 years of age for men is 168 per minute and that for women is 159 per minute.

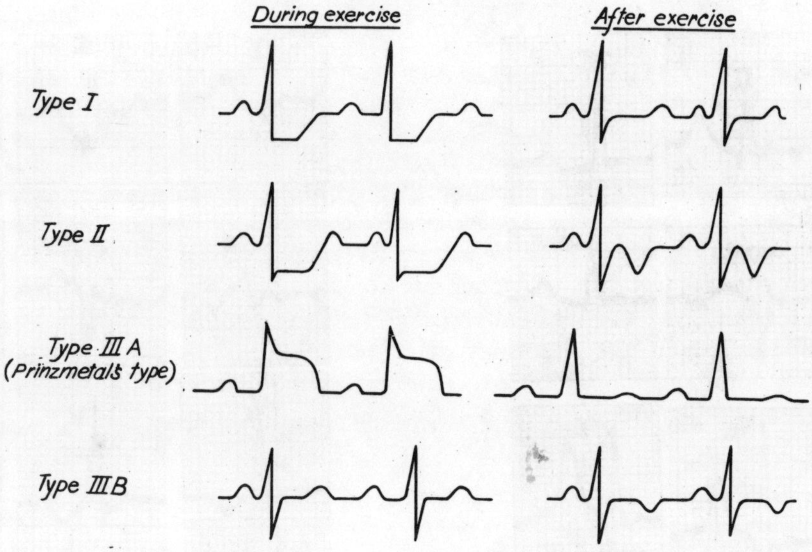

Fig. 48. Diagrammatic representation of types of S-T segment displacement *during exercise* and 1 *minute after exercise*

Exercise testing is contraindicated in impending, acute or healing myocardial infarction, unstable angina pectoris, tight aortic stenosis, heart failure, moderate and severe hypertension, uncontrolled cardiac arrhythmias and any other acute systemic illness.

The Holter technique of ambulatory electrocardiographic recording is very useful for detecting intermittent cardiac arrhythmias, conduction defects, pre-excitation syndromes, sick sinus syndromes, long Q-T syndromes etc. The patient uses a light portable tape recorder for continuous electrocardiographic recordings for 24 hours or more during his daily activities. The patient also records any symptom during the Holter monitoring operation in a diary. Electrocardiographic recordings would demonstrate cardiac arrhythmias which may develop during exertion, emotions, excitement, sleep etc. and help to outline the method of treatment of the patient and evaluate the effects of therapy.

The next method of detecting myocardial ischaemia, conduction defects, and sinus node dysfunction which occur intermittently and irregularly, is by *teletransmission of electrocardiographic recordings.* As these disturbances do not occur daily Holter technique often fails to detect such disturbances. These arrhythmias, and disturbances of origin and conduction of the pacemaker impulses can be recorded by teletransmission of electrocardiographic tracings by the patient himself who had been trained adequately for the same. When symptoms appears the patient calls the receiving unit over the telephone, applies the electrodes on his person as per previous training and transmits his electrocardiographic tracing to the receiving unit. After getting the electrocardiographic tracings the receiving unit sends messages to the attending physician who analyses the electrocardiograms and sends proper instructions to the patient to manage the disturbing rhythm. For the correct operation of the equipments the patients must be adequately trained.

In case of angina pectoris with a normal electrocardiogram, an electrocardiographic tracing taken after tachycardia produced by atrial pacing may show abnormal findings in it.

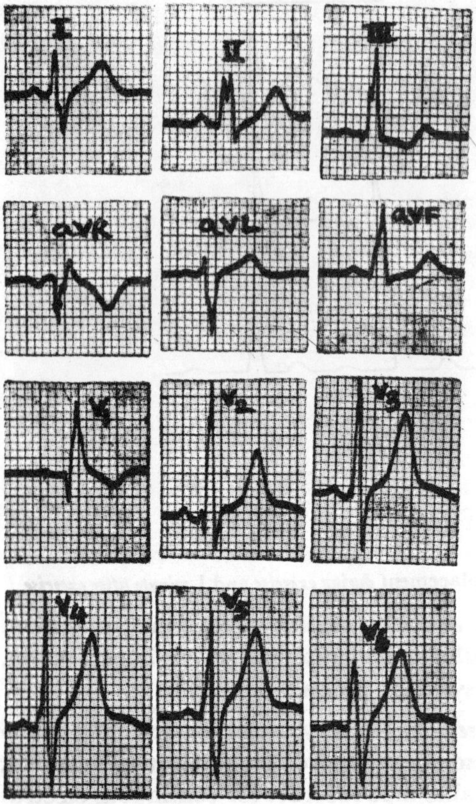

Fig. 49–A.

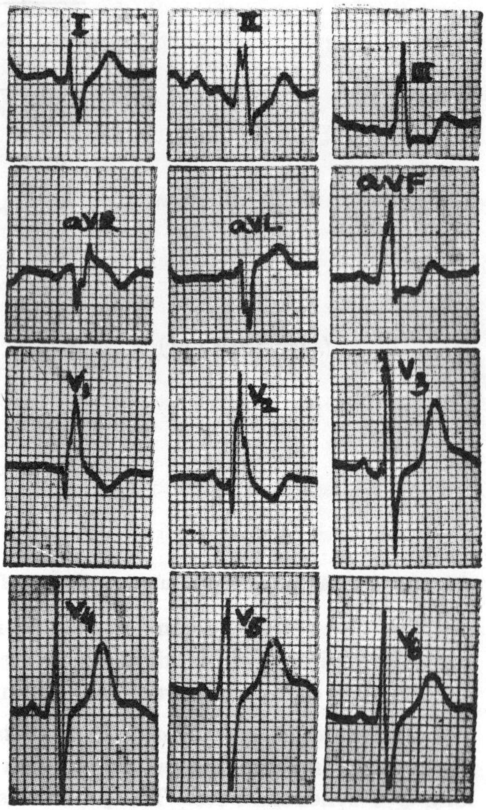

Fig. 49–B.

Fig. 49–A is a tracing before exercise from a person who had no symptoms. Fig. 49–B is a tracing after exercise showing S–T segment depression and T wave changes. There is also right bundle-branch block. An aberrant ventricular conduction is seen in lead V_2.

Electrocardiographic studies after atrial pacing

Effects of tachycardia produced artificially by atrial pacing may be studied on the electrocardiogram of persons without any symptom of coronary artery disease. An intra-cardiac electrode catheter is introduced through a forearm vein into the right atrium so that the catheter tip lies near the opening of the superior vena cava. As the pacing rate is increased gradually in stages by controlling the artificial pacemaker atrial capture is obtained; when the atrial pacing rate is on an average of 124 minute anginal pain, S–T segment depression or atrioventricular block may appear thereby revealing an occult coronary artery disease. The occurrence of chest pain is an indication to stop atrial pacing.

CHAPTER VI

THE ARRHYTHMIAS

The term arrhythmia indicates absence of a normal rhythm and is used when the intervals in between the successive QRS complexes are unequal or when the cardiac excitations take place at an abnormal rate from the S–A node or when they originate from a focus other than the S–A node.

Arrhythmia may arise when there is either a defect in the impulse formation or a defect in the impulse conduction.

A. Arrhythmias arising out of defective impulse formation may be as follows:

1. Sinus Arrhythmia.
2. Sinus Tachycardia.
3. Sinus Bradycardia.
4. Escape–Capture Bigeminy.
5. Ectopic Beat.
6. Sino-Atrial Block and Sinus Arrest.
7. Atrial Flutter.
8. Atrial Fibrillation.
9. Atrial Flutter-Fibrillation.
10. A–V Nodal Rhythm.
11. Reciprocal Rhythm.
12. Paroxysmal Supraventricular Tachycardia.
13. Paroxysmal Ventricular Tachycardia.
14. Coupled Beats.
15. Ventricular Fibrillation.
16. Dual Rhythm.
17. Wandering Pacemaker.
18. Parasystole.
19. Summation Beat (Fusion Beat or Dressler Beat).
20. Interference Dissociation and Interference Beat (Ventricular Capture).

B. Arrhythmias arising out of defective impulse conduction may be as follows (*vide* Conduction Defects):

1. Wolff-Parkinson-White Syndrome.
2. Heart Block.

Sinus Arrhythmia

Irregularity in rhythm may occur physiologically due to the presence of sinus arrhythmia and it is recognised by the presence of absolutely normal P–QRS–T complex, P–R interval, Q–T duration, and S–T segment with an intermittent shortening and lengthening of the intervals in between the P–QRS–T complexes. The heart rate increases during inspiration and slows down during expiration. Rarely this may not have any relation to respiration (Fig. 50).

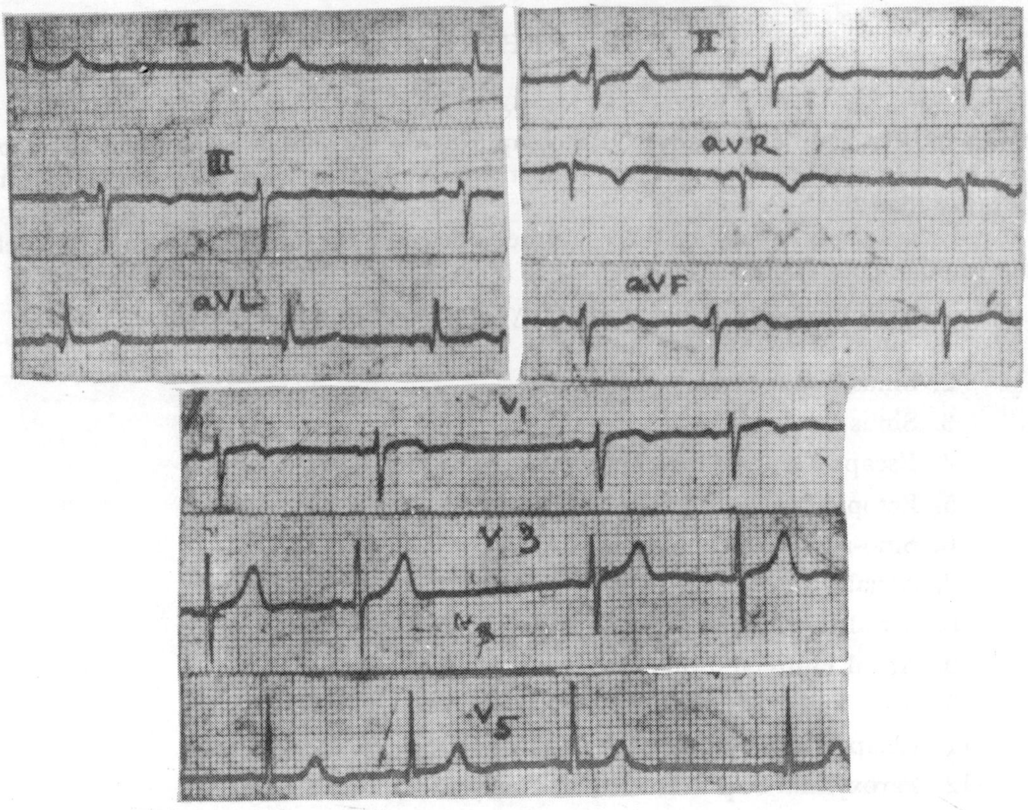

Fig. 50.

Fig. 50 is an electrocardiogram showing typical features of sinus arrhythmia.

Sinus Tachycardia

This is said to be present when there is tachycardia (heart rate more than 100/minute) with excitatory impulses coming from the S–A node so that the P waves and P–R intervals are normal in absence of atrial enlargement and accelerated conduction. This is found after exertion, emotion, excitement, rheumatic fever, and infections such as tuberculosis, diphtheria, etc. This may sometimes be confused with paroxysmal atrial tachycardia which may be diagnosed by a constant R–R interval, an abrupt slowing of heart rate during carotid sinus pressure, termination of tachycardia after carotid sinus pressure in some cases and a difference in the pattern of atrial complexes during and after carotid sinus pressure.

Sinus Bradycardia

This is said to be present when there is bradycardia (heart rate less than 60/minute) in presence of absolutely normal P waves and P–R intervals. This is found in athletes, in some normal persons, in myxoedema, obstructive jaundice, etc. (Fig. 51).

Escape-Capture Bigeminy

In escape-capture bigeminy or pseudoreciprocal rhythm there is an upright P wave between the two QRS complexes of the coupled beats. The upright P wave and the long P–R interval indicate its origin from the S–A node and conduction defect in the A–V

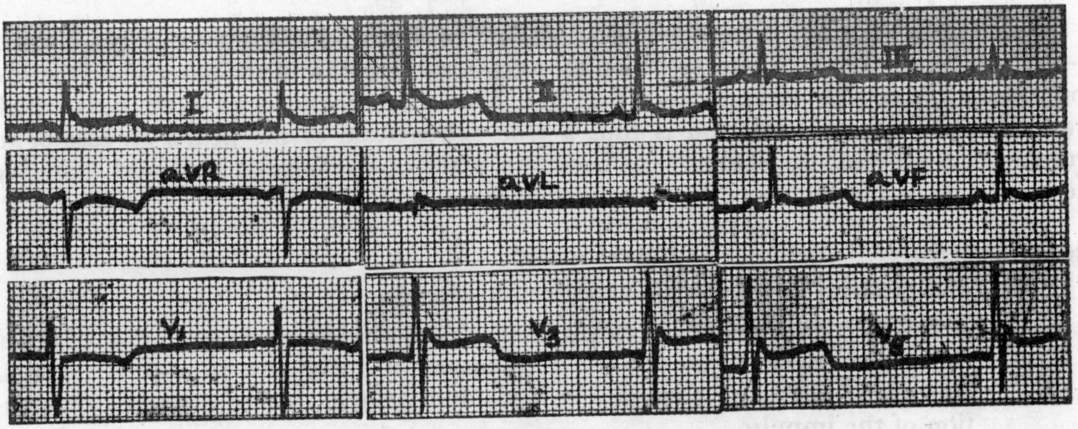

Fig. 51.
Fig. 51 is an electrocardiogram having sinus bradycardia.

node respectively. The condition develops when there is an irregular sinus bradycardia intercepted by nodal escape beats with retrograde A–V nodal block.

Ectopic or Premature Beat

Ectopic beat will produce an ectopic QRS complex among a series of regular QRS complexes resulting from normal excitations from S–A node. An ectopic QRS complex originates from an excitatory focus other than the S–A node and is identified by a small pause before it and a long pause after it.

When the sumtotal of the small pause (R–R interval) and the long pause is equal to two normal pauses (i.e., two normal R–R intervals) in the tracing, it is said to be fully compensatory; this occurs in ventricular ectopic beat.

When the sumtotal of the small and long pauses is less than two normal pauses in the tracing, it is said to be an incomplete compensatory pause; this occurs in atrial and nodal ectopic beat.

The QRS complex of the ectopic beat may be of normal or bizarre pattern, depending on the site of origin of the ectopic beat. The bizarre pattern is seen in ventricular ectopic beat.

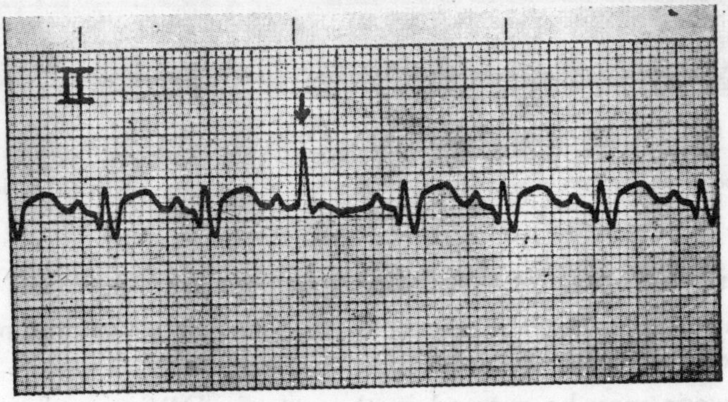

Fig. 52.
Fig. 52 shows an electrocardiographic tracing with an interpolated atrial ectopic beat (extrasystole).

Sometimes when an ectopic complex occurs in the midway between two normal P–QRS–T complexes, it is said to be *an interpolated ectopic beat* and the pauses both before and after it are smaller than normal (Fig. 52). This actually causes an extra beat which is added to the normal beats and is thus a true extrasystole of the heart. In case of an ordinary ectopic beat, the ectopic beat occurs in place of one normal beat and therefore the heart rate is not increased by its occurrence.

Atrial ectopic beat

The characteristic features of an atrial ectopic beat are:

1. The QRS complex of the ectopic beat is similar in appearance to that of other beats in that lead, provided the conduction of excitatory impulse is normal. Rarely the QRS complex may be wide and bizarre due to aberrant conduction of the impulse.
2. The P wave preceding the ectopic QRS complex is not similar to other P waves in that lead.
3. The P–R interval of the ectopic P–QRS–T complex is usually shorter than that of other P–QRS–T complexes. Rarely the P–R interval of the ectopic complex may be equal to or even greater than that of a normal P–QRS–T complex in the same tracing. This depends on the site of origin of the ectopic focus in the atrial wall.

Blocked atrial ectopic beat

When an atrial ectopic beat occurs very early it may not be followed by a ventricular complex as the myocardium is still in the refractory phase. Such an ectopic beat is called a blocked atrial ectopic beat which may occur singly or sometimes alternately giving rise to an atrial bigeminal rhythm, i.e., a normal sinus beat is regularly followed by a blocked atrial beat (Fig. 53).

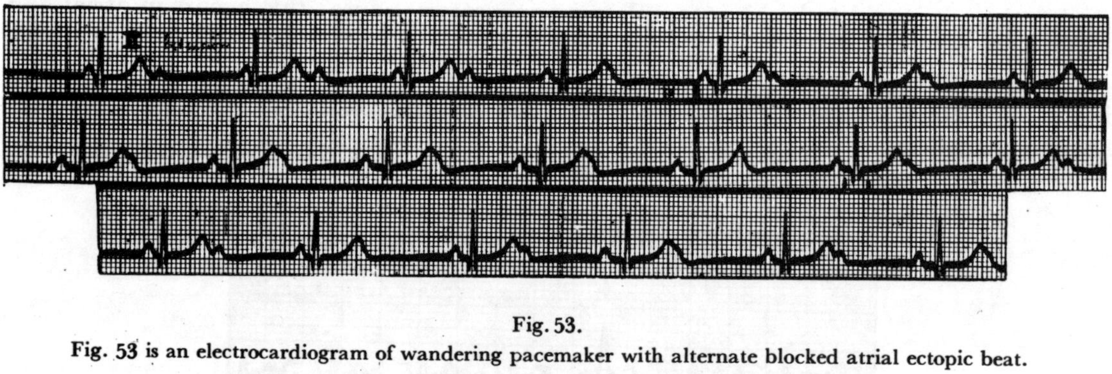

Fig. 53.

Fig. 53 is an electrocardiogram of wandering pacemaker with alternate blocked atrial ectopic beat.

Nodal ectopic beat

The characteristic features of a nodal ectopic beat are:

1. The shape and size of the ectopic QRS complex are usually normal and similar to that of other QRS complexes.
2. The P wave may be merged in the ectopic QRS complex or may be visible before or after it, depending on the exact site of origin of the ectopic beat in the A–V node; and when visible the P wave may be inverted or deformed.

Ventricular ectopic beat

This is recognised by the following features (Fig. 54):

1. A bizarre pattern of the ectopic QRS complex.
2. The ectopic QRS complex is not preceded by a P wave.
3. The T wave is directed opposite to that of the main deflection of the ectopic QRS complex.

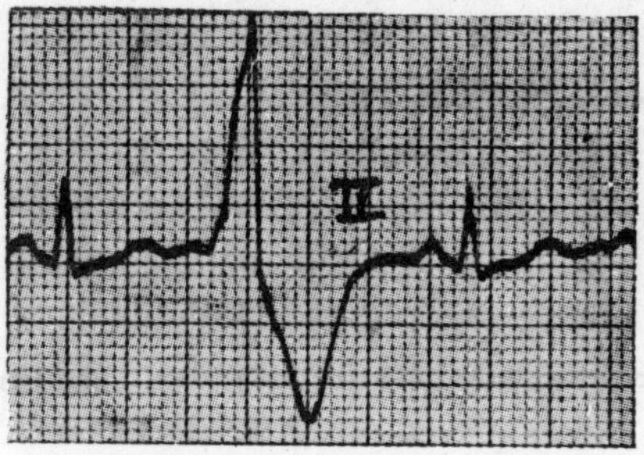

Fig. 54.

Fig. 54 is an electrocardiographic tracing having a ventricular ectopic beat.

Main-Stem extrasystole.

When the ectopic beat occurs from an ectopic focus situated in the main stem of the bundle of His, the QRS complex is similar to a supraventricular beat but the compensatory pause in this case is complete (full).

ESCAPE BEATS

Apart from the S-A node which serves as the normal natural pace-maker of the heart, hundreds of "extra" or "reserve" or "demand" or "substitute" or "standby" pace-makers are situated in the sub-endocardial layers of the heart in the atrial, A-V nodal or ventricular tissues of the cardiac apparatus. As a life-saving measure one of these foci of specialised tissue is called into play which fires an excitation wave causing an effective ventricular beat when the normal excitation wave fails to originate from the S-A node.

When the S-A node is normally active the reserve pace-makers are suppressed as they are discharged before they could build up to the 'firing level'. When the S-A node is inactive the reserve pace-maker is no longer discharged earlier giving it a chance to reach the firing level. Thus the reserve pace-maker gets a chance to fire and originate an excitation wave giving rise to a ventricular contraction. The ventricular beat thus occurring, is known as an "escape beat" or a "postmature beat."

An excitation wave which occurs as a result of cardiac irritability, originates in spite of normal activity of S-A node and gives rise to a ventricular beat earlier than when it is due. This is called a premature or ectopic or extrasystolic beat which serves no useful purpose. This must

be differentiated from an "escape beat" which occurs much later than when a ventricular beat is due and is a life-saving process (vide figure 55).

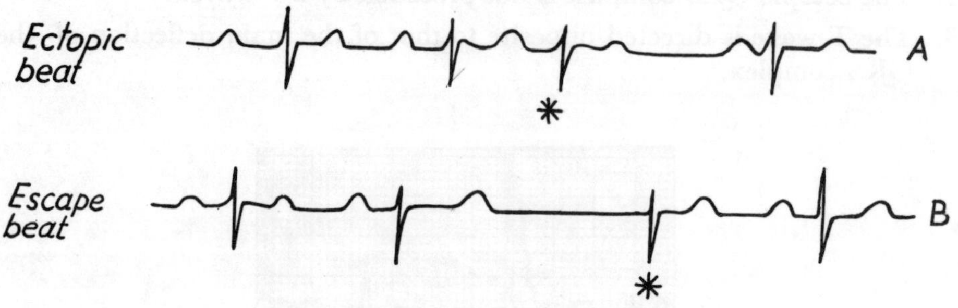

Fig. 55 Diagrammatic representation of an ectopic beat (A) and an escape beat (B).

Sustained ectopic beats from a focus of excitation cause 'paroxysmal tachycardias' which are not usually helpful for the subject.

Sustained escape beats are slower in rate, rate of firing being in the slow to normal range of the heart rate and is absolutely physiological and should never be suppressed. The slow, regular rhythm that follows is designated as idio-atrial, idio-nodal or idio-ventricular rhythm according to the location of the reserve pace-maker in the atrial, A-V nodal or ventricular tissues respectively.

Sino-Atrial Block and Sinus Arrest

S-A block is indicated by the absence of the P-QRS-T complexes at the expected time of their appearance due to failure of the sinus node to originate an impulse. Thus there will be a long pause in between the two normal P-QRS-T complexes which is usually equal to the summation of two or more normal P-P intervals (Figs. 56 & 57). The long interval may be interrupted by a QRS complex arising out of an excitatory focus from other sites of the heart; this abnormal beat is called an 'Escape Beat'; in such a case the term 'sinus arrest' is preferred.

When this escape beat originates from an ectopic focus situated in the atrial wall or in the A—V node it is called an atrial escape or a nodal escape respectively; and when the focus is situated in the ventricular muscle, it is called a ventricular escape.

Usually a single beat is dropped at a time. But if the sinus node fails to resume its functions for a long period the A-V node or the ventricle may serve as a temporary pacemaker of the heart. The first beat after resumption of the sinus rhythm may have aberrant conduction.

The sinus arrest and atrial standstill may occur after carotid sinus stimulation, quinidine or digitalis administration and in heart disease involving sinus node such as rheumatic fever, myocardial infarction, etc.

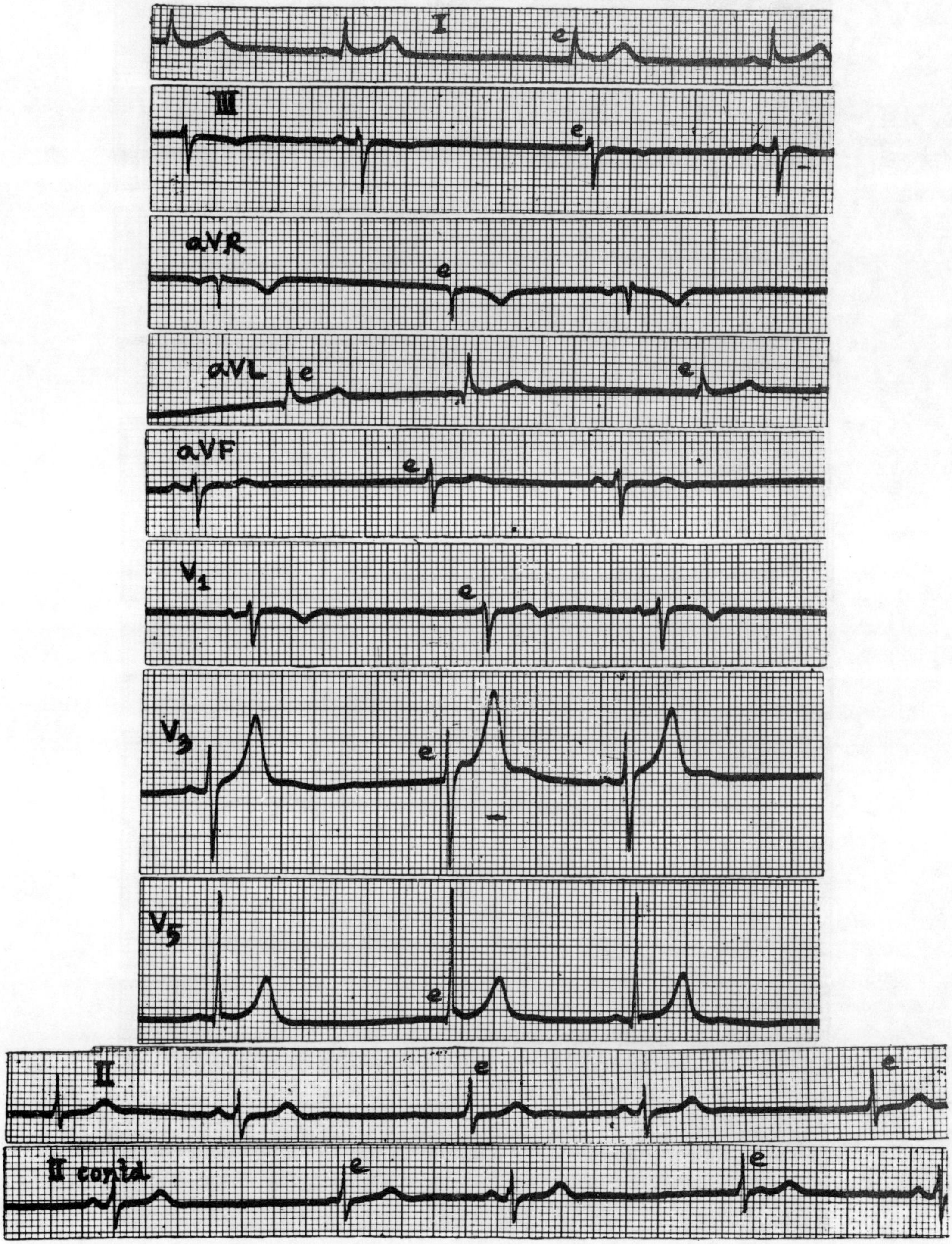

Fig. 56.

Fig. 56 shows a tracing of sinus arrest followed by nodal escape.

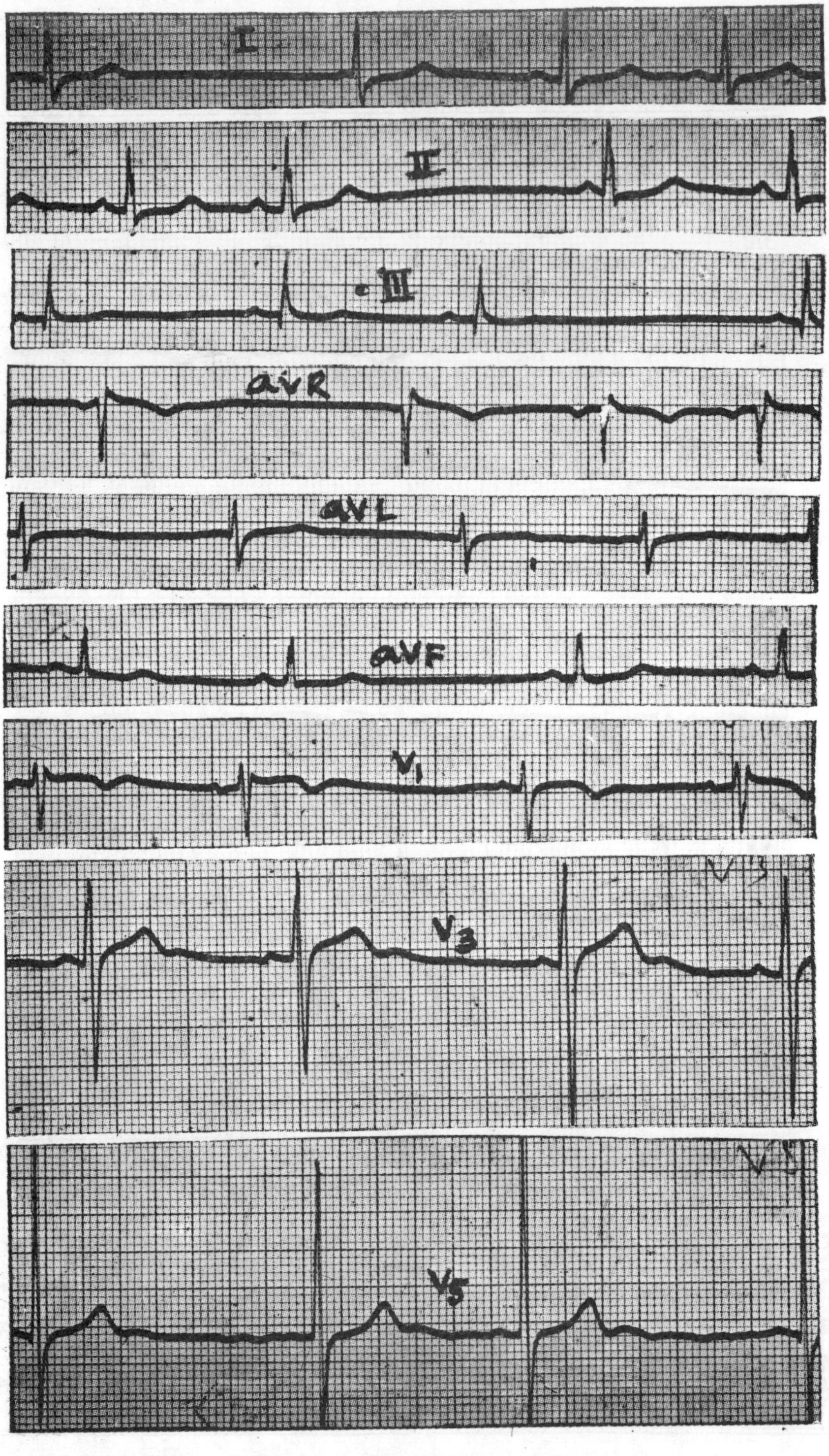

Fig. 57.

Fig. 57 is an electrocardiographic tracing of both S–A block and sinus arrest. In leads I, aVR, V_1 and V_5 there is sinus arrest followed by nodal escape. In the rest there is intermittent S–A block.

Idionodal and Idioventricular rhythm

In case of complete S–A block there is cardiac standstill which may continue till the ventricles are activated by an ectopic focus; when this excitable focus is situated in the A–V node, and emits impulses slowly at a regular rhythm, it is called idionodal rhythm; the QRS complex in such a case is of normal duration as that of a sinus beat.

When the excitable focus is situated in a ventricle and emits impulses regularly and usually at a slower rate, it is called idioventricular rhythm; this commonly occurs in complete A–V nodal block. Here the QRS complex is wider than that of the normal sinus beat.

Atrial Flutter

This is recognised by:

1. Presence of flutter waves which assume the garden-brick or saw-tooth appearance in the electrocardiographic tracing, the atrial rate usually varying from 250 to 350/min.
2. Absence of an isoelectric base line after the end of the P wave and before the beginning of the corresponding QRS complex.

Atrial flutter may occur, with a regular or an irregular ventricular rhythm.

A. *With a regular ventricular rhythm*

This occurs as a result of a fixed atrioventricular relationship such as 4 : 1, 3 : 1, etc.; thus in case of 4 : 1 A–V relationship, for every 4 atrial contractions (P wave) there is one ventricular contraction (QRS complex) regularly throughout that particular tracing (Fig. 58).

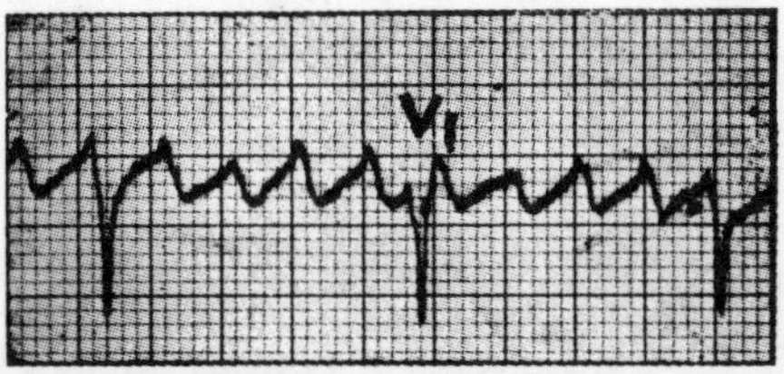

Fig. 58.
Fig. 58 shows a tracing of atrial flutter with a regular ventricular rhythm.

B. *With an irregular ventricular rhythm*

This occurs as a result of varying atrioventricular relationship. In this case the ventricular complexes (QRS complexes) are seen after 3, 4, or more atrial contractions (P waves) in an irregular fashion (Fig. 59) in the same tracing.

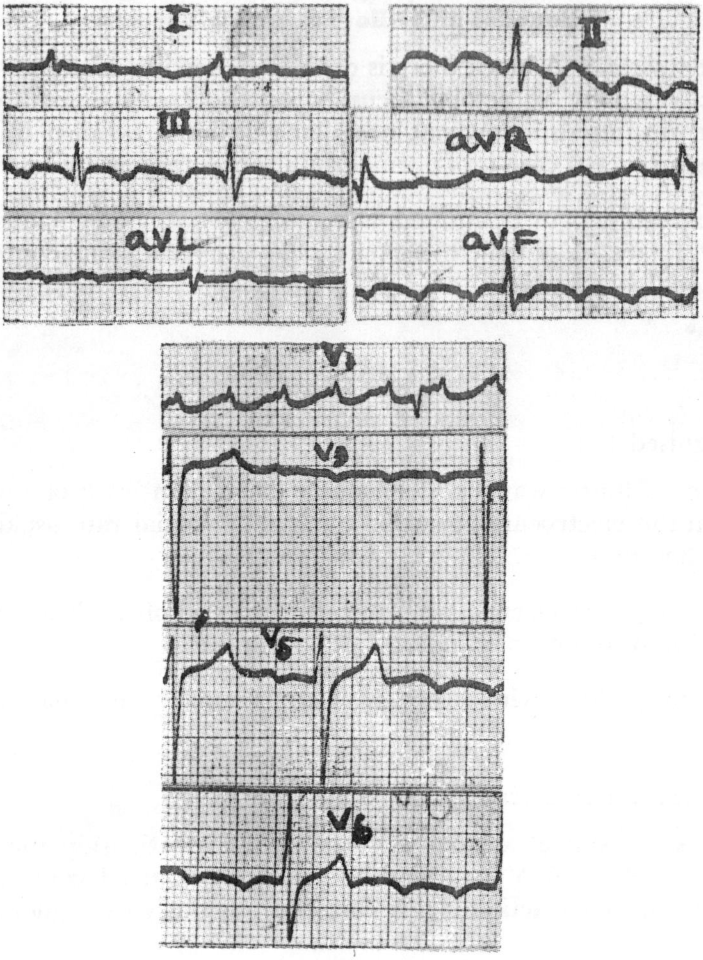

Fig. 59.

Fig. 59 is an electrocardiogram of atrial flutter with an irregular ventricular rhythm due to varying degrees of heart block.

Atrial Fibrillation

This is diagnosed by (Figs. 60, 61 & 62):

1. Irregular placing of the QRS complexes.
2. Absence of regular P waves.
3. Presence of fibrillary or 'f' waves which are best seen in lead V_1. The atrial rate is calculated by dividing 1500 by the number of small squares lying in between the peaks (crests) of the two successive 'f' waves. Sometimes the fibrillary waves may not be visible in the tracing.

The average ventricular rate is calculated from the mean value of the shortest and the longest intervals between two successive ventricular complexes.

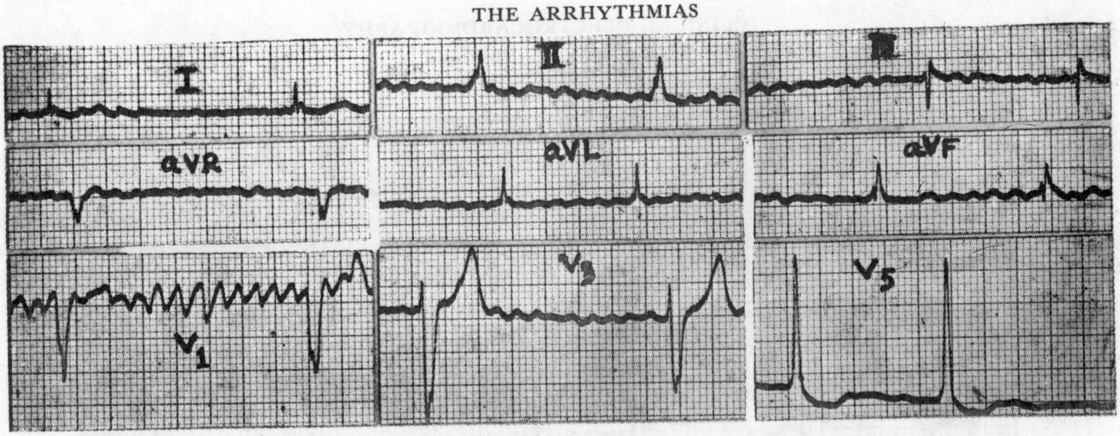

Fig. 60.
Fig. 60 is an electrocardiogram showing atrial fibrillation in a patient aged 52 years suffering from ischaemic heart disease.

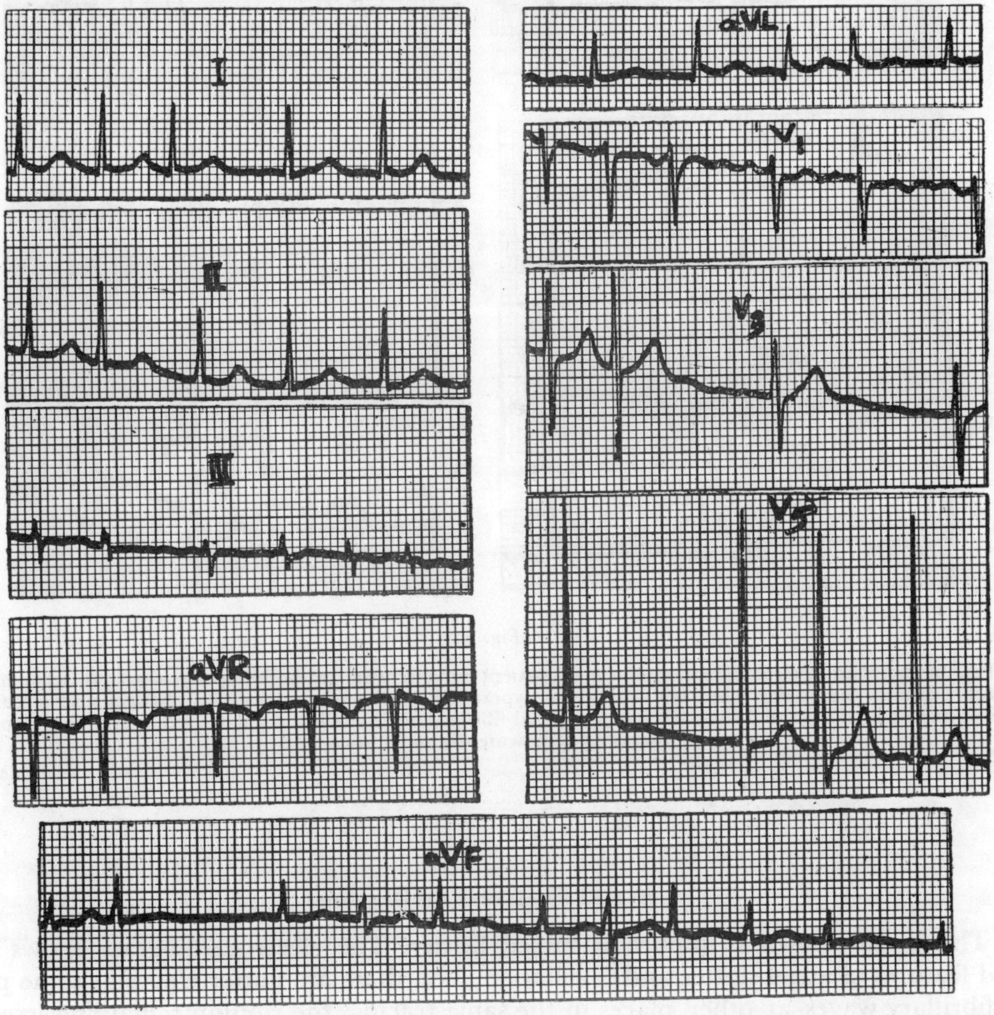

Fig. 61.
Fig. 61 is an electrocardiogram of a case of cardiomyopathy showing atrial fibrillation and left ventricular hypertrophy. There is hardly visible 'f' waves.

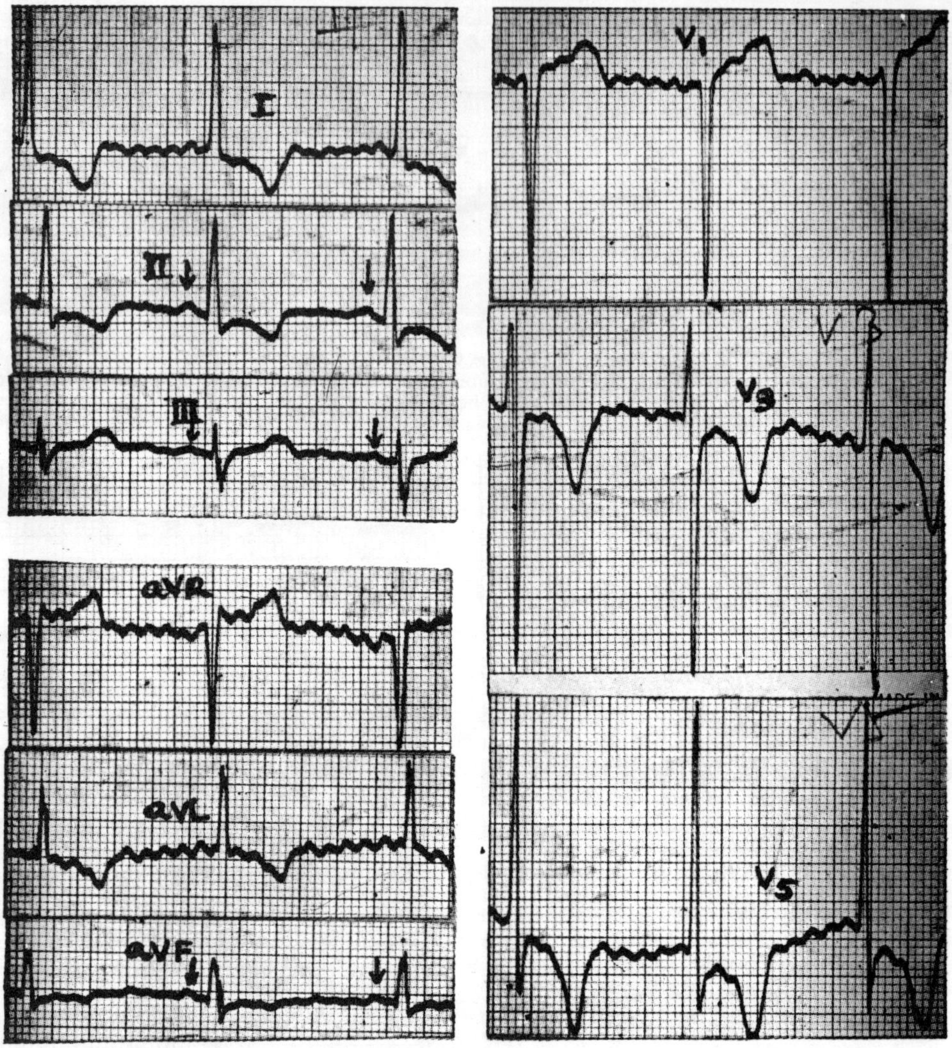

Fig. 62.

Fig. 62 shows an electrocardiogram of a male patient aged 62 who had both hypertension and ischaemic heart disease; the tracing shows left ventricular hypertrophy, ischaemic myocardial changes and a base line having artefacts simulating 'f' waves of atrial fibrillation; there is a regular rhythm and the arrow marks (↓) indicate distinct P waves.

Atrial Flutter-Fibrillation

This is also known as impure or mixed flutter. The electrocardiogram shows combined features of atrial flutter and fibrillation, i.e., there are flutter waves at some places and fibrillary waves at other places in the same tracing, the rhythm remaining irregular (Fig. 63).

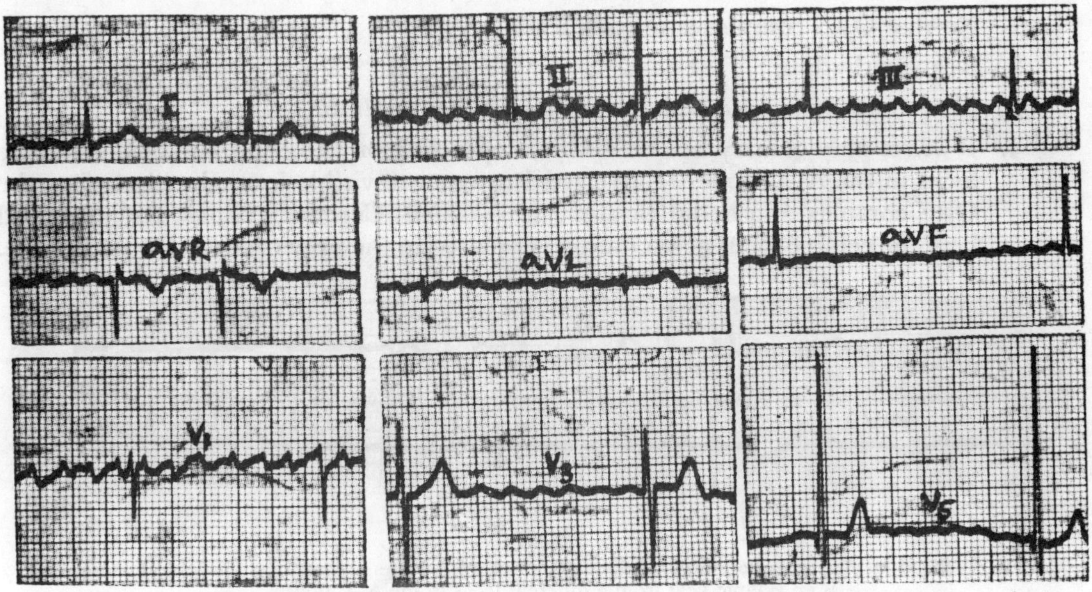

Fig. 63.

Fig. 63 shows a tracing of mixed atrial flutter and fibrillation.

A–V Nodal Rhythm

If there is depression of the sinoatrial node due to any cause, the A–V node may function as the pacemaker and the rhythm which arises out of it is called the nodal rhythm. This is recognised by (Figs. 64 & 65):

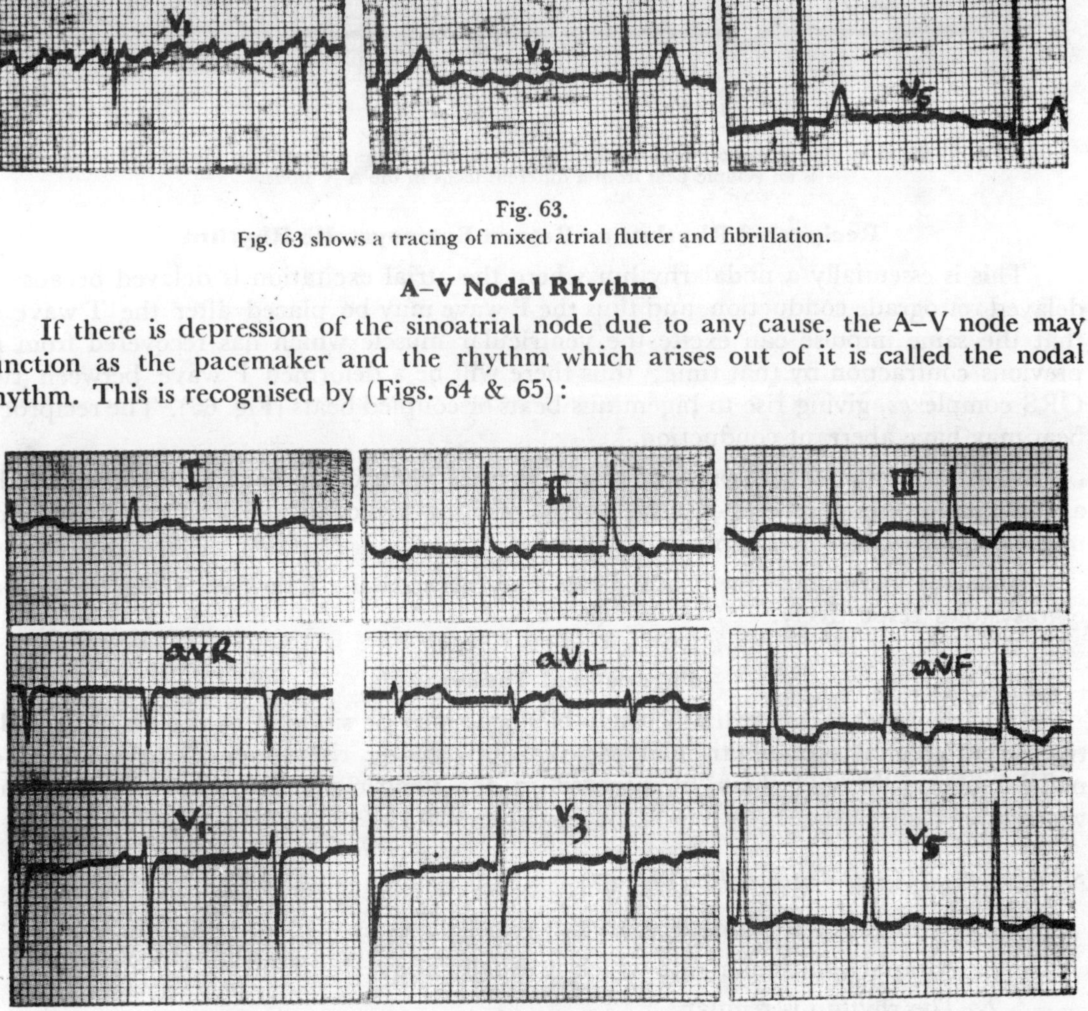

Fig. 64.

Fig. 64 is an electrocardiogram of intermittent nodal rhythm showing P waves occurring after the QRS complexes which indicate that the excitatory focus is situated in the lower part of the A–V node; leads V_1, V_3 & V_5 show a return of the sinus rhythm.

1. Normal QRS complexes in each lead.
2. Regular rhythm.
3. Slow ventricular rate which is usually around 60/min.
4. P waves may or may not be visible, depending on the exact site of the ectopic focus in the A–V node. If inverted P waves are visible immediately before the QRS complexes in nodal rhythm, it is called Coronary Sinus Rhythm and here the ectopic focus of excitation is situated in the upper part of the A–V node.

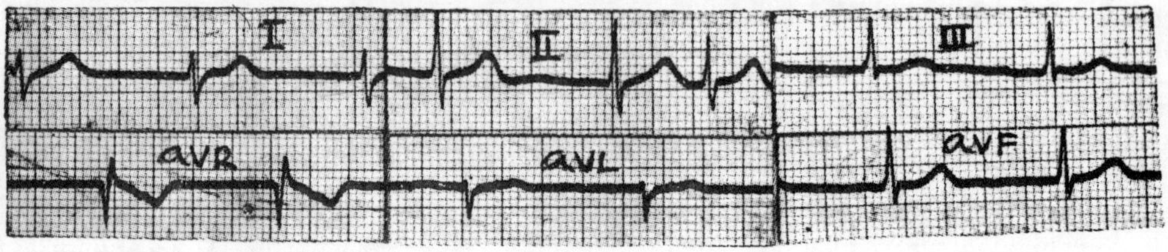

Fig. 65.

Fig. 65 shows an electrocardiogram of nodal rhythm where P waves are not seen: in lead II there is an ectopic beat from a different focus in the A–V node.

Reciprocal Rhythm or Return Extrasystolic Rhythm

This is essentially a nodal rhythm where the atrial excitation is delayed because of delayed retrograde conduction, and thus the P wave may be placed after the T wave so that the same impulse can excite the ventricular muscle which has recovered from its previous contraction by that time; thus there will be a deformed P wave between two QRS complexes, giving rise to bigeminus beats or coupled beats (Fig. 66). The reciprocal beat may have aberrant conduction.

Very rarely the excitation from the reciprocal ventricular beat may return to the atrial muscle through the A–V node again, eliciting a second atrial contraction which may be followed by a 3rd ventricular response.

Atrial or ventricular reciprocal beats may occasionally follow atrial or ventricular extrasystoles respectively.

Paroxysmal Tachycardia

In paroxysmal tachycardia the excitable focus may be situated in the atrial or nodal tissue (paroxysmal supraventricular tachycardia), giving rise to paroxysmal atrial or nodal tachycardia or it may be situated in the ventricle giving rise to paroxysmal ventricular tachycardia.

A. *Paroxysmal Atrial Tachycardia* (Fig. 67)

The characteristic features of atrial tachycardia are:

1. A rapid ventricular rate which is usually above 160/min.
2. The rhythm is regular.
3. The P waves are usually visible before the QRS complexes and the P–R intervals are usually shortened.
4. The QRS duration is normal.

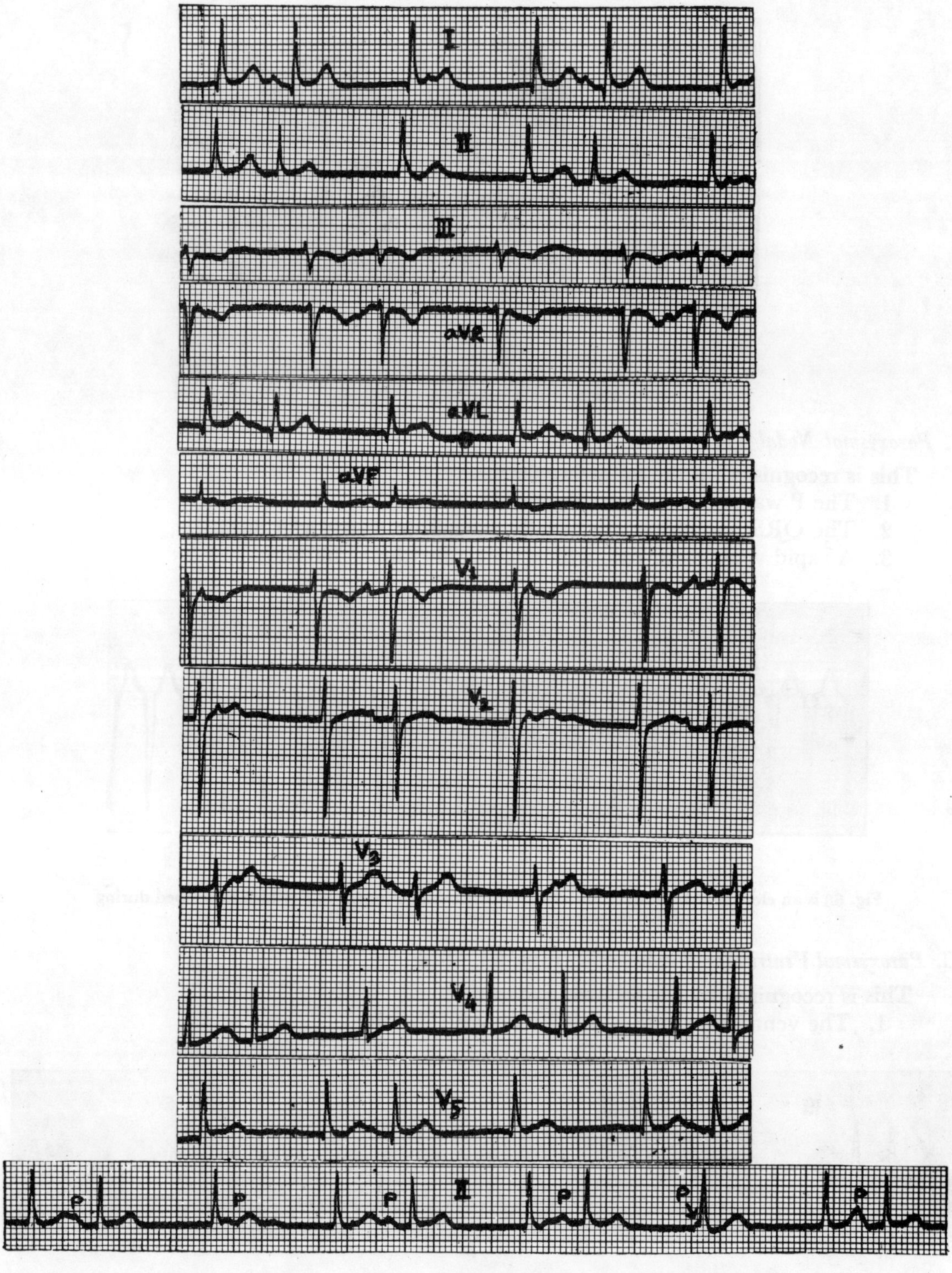

Fig. 66.

Fig. 66 is an electrocardiogram of reciprocal rhythm with delayed retrograde conduction through the A–V node.

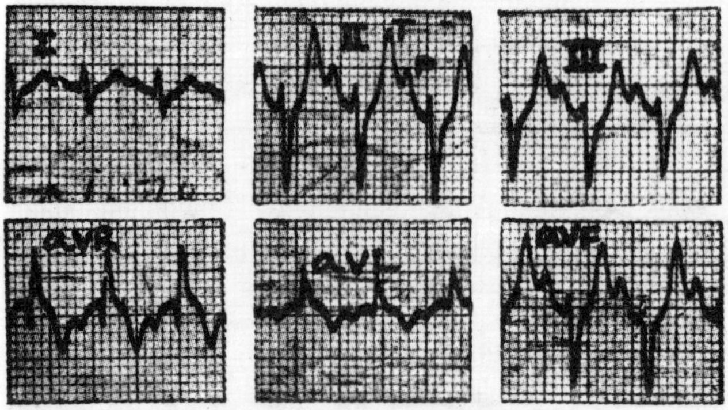

Fig. 67.

Fig. 67 shows an electrocardiogram of paroxysmal atrial tachycardia with a heart rate of 176/min.

B. *Paroxysmal Nodal Tachycardia* (Fig. 68)

This is recognised by the following features:

1. The P waves are not usually visible.
2. The QRS complexes are usually normal in shape and duration.
3. A rapid ventricular rate which is usually above 160/min.

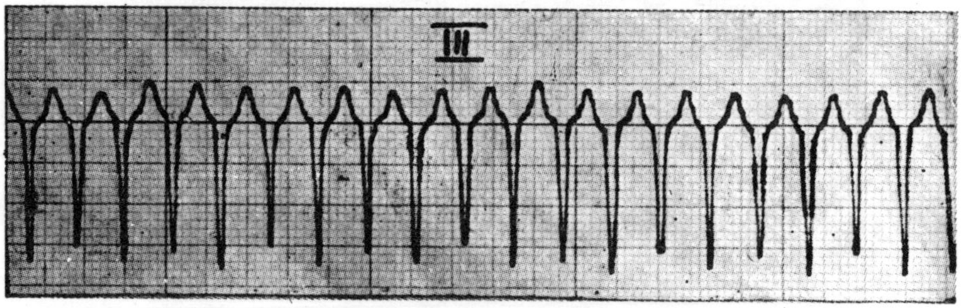

Fig. 68.

Fig. 68 is an electrocardiogram of nodal tachycardia (supraventricular) which developed during cardiac catheterisation. The heart rate is 250/min.

C. *Paroxysmal Ventricular Tachycardia* (Figs. 69, 70 & 71)

This is recognised by the following features:

1. The ventricular rate is usually above 160/min.

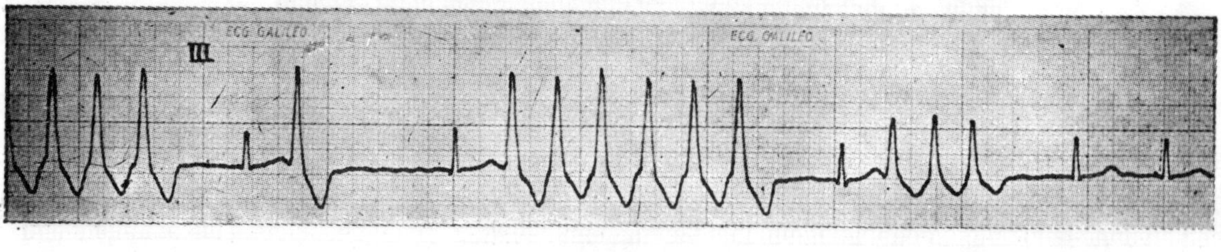

Fig. 69.

Fig. 69 is an electrocardiogram of intermittent paroxysmal ventricular tachycardia obtained during cardiac catheterisation.

2. The QRS complexes are wider and are of bizarre pattern.
3. There may be slightly irregular rhythm.
4. The P waves may occasionally be visible.

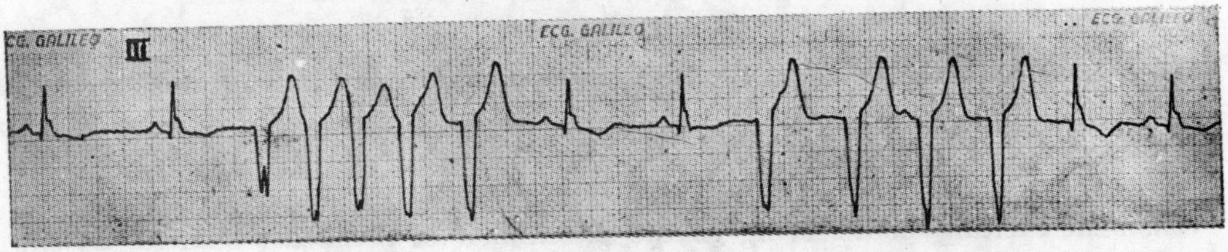

Fig. 70.

Fig. 70 is an electrocardiogram of intermittent paroxysmal ventricular tachycardia intervened by sinus rhythm obtained during cardiac catheterisation; immediately after the second paroxysm there is a nodal beat followed by sinus rhythm.

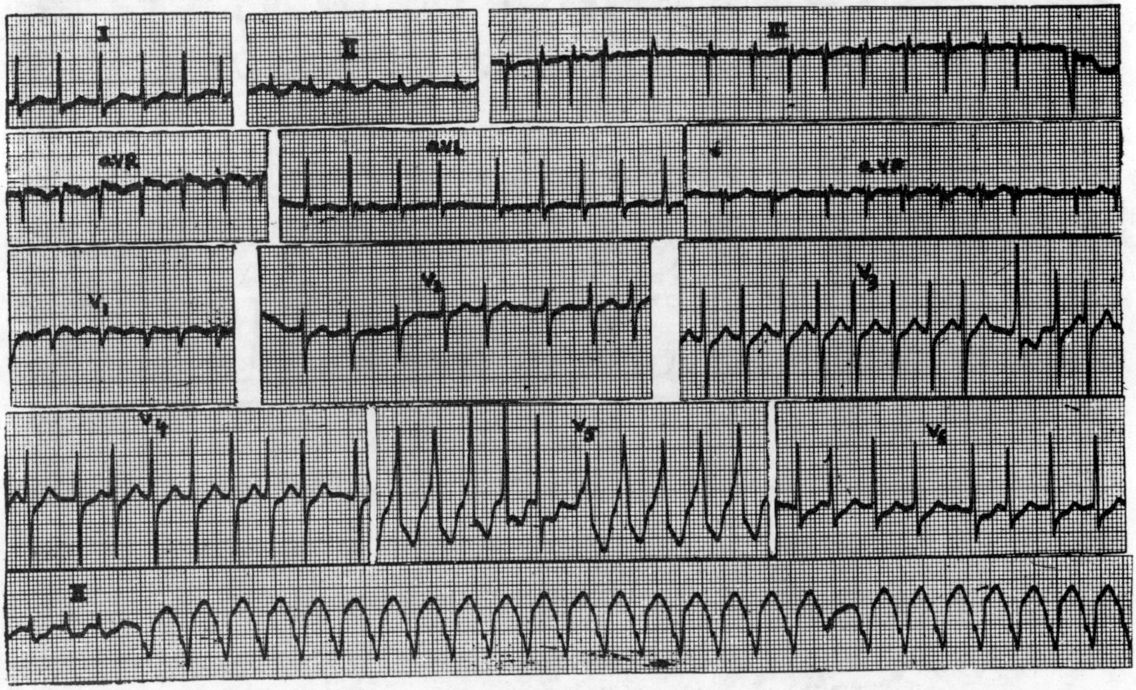

Fig. 71.

Fig. 71 presents an electrocardiogram of a male patient aged 62 years who had ischaemic heart disease with atrial fibrillation; he developed intermittent paroxysmal ventricular tachycardia and ultimately died. A bizarre QRS complex shown in the bottom strip is a Dressler beat.

Coupled Beats

Coupled beats are recognised by the occurrence of ventricular complexes in pairs and may develop in the electrocardiographic tracing under the following conditions:

1. When every alternate beat is an ectopic beat.
2. When there is 3 : 2 A–V heart block.
3. When there is a reciprocal rhythm.

Ventricular Fibrillation

In ventricular fibrillation the electrocardiographic tracing shows no P waves and the QRS complexes are wide and biphasic without any identifiable Q wave or T wave.

Dual Rhythm

When both the S–A node and the A–V node emit impulses and stimulate ventricles irregularly with variable asynchronism the rhythm may be designated as Dual Rhythm.

Wandering Pacemaker

When the exciting focus serving as the pacemaker of the heart changes its site of origin from the sinus node to the A–V node or atrial wall, the pacemaker is then described as the wandering pacemaker. Here the shape of the P wave and the P–R intervals alter from beat to beat. The rhythm, however, is usually regular (Fig. 72).

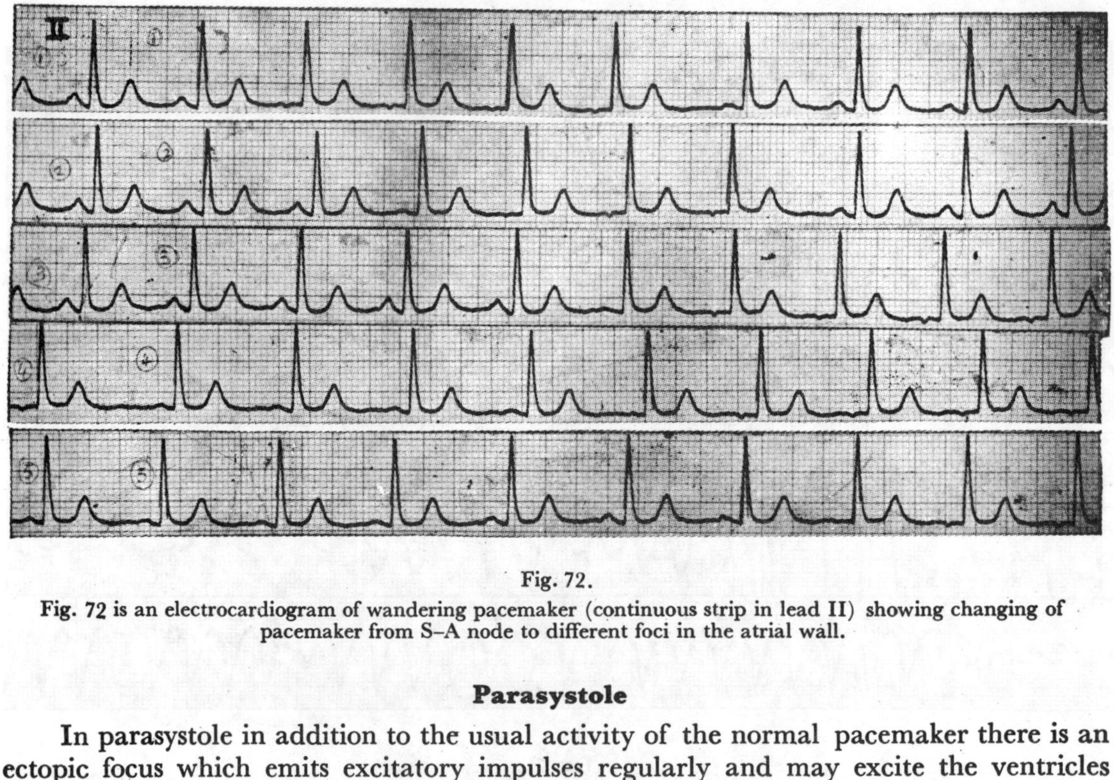

Fig. 72.

Fig. 72 is an electrocardiogram of wandering pacemaker (continuous strip in lead II) showing changing of pacemaker from S–A node to different foci in the atrial wall.

Parasystole

In parasystole in addition to the usual activity of the normal pacemaker there is an ectopic focus which emits excitatory impulses regularly and may excite the ventricles whenever they reach the ventricles outside their refractory phase. This ectopic focus is not depolarised by the normal excitatory impulse from the pacemaker of the heart probably due to the presence of a region of depressed conduction, or local block at the site of the ectopic focus. This region of so-called electrophysiological isolation is uninfluenced by factors influencing the S–A node.

Summation Beats (Fusion Beats and Dressler Beats)

In this type of abnormal beat the resulting QRS complex is wide and bizarre as the ventricles are partly stimulated by a normal sinus impulse, and partly by an ectopic focus which is mostly ventricular in origin which emits an impulse late in diastole. Thus the ventricles are more or less simultaneously stimulated from two sources and the beat that follows is called a fusion beat. The fusion beat may also occur if there are two ventricular ectopic pacemakers competing for the control of the ventricles.

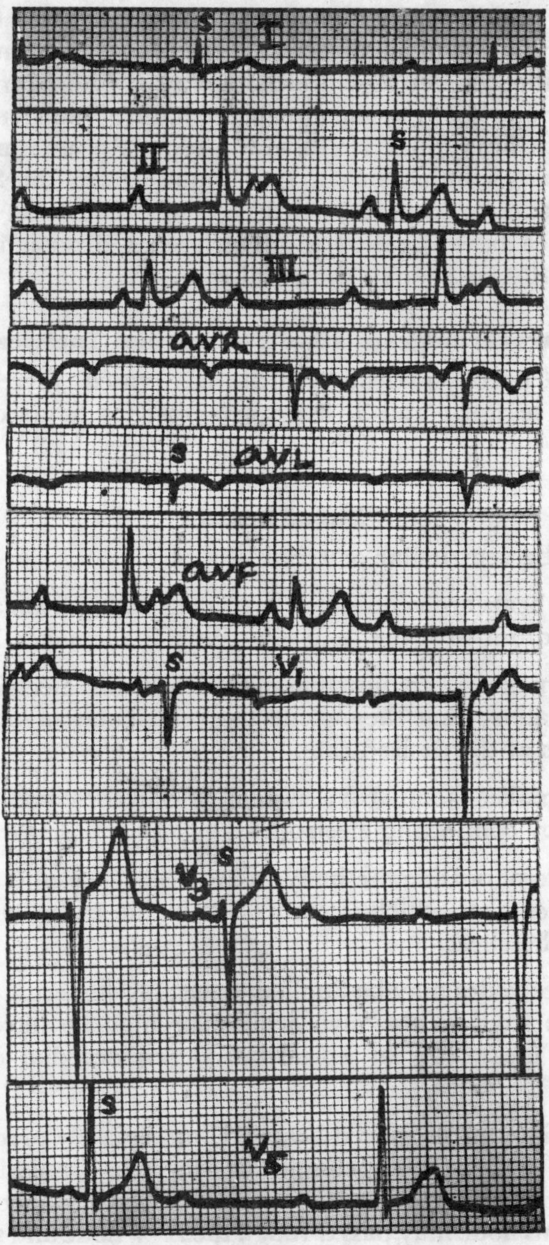

Fig. 73.

Fig. 73 is an electrocardiogram of complete heart block with idionodal rhythm; the QRS complexes marked 'S' are sinus beats and thus these are 'ventricular captures' where excitations from S–A node were able to pass through the A–V node and stimulate the ventricles.

In paroxysmal ventricular tachycardia fusion beat may occur due to excitation of the ventricles from an ectopic ventricular focus other than that causing ventricular tachycardia and the fusion beat that follows is called a Dressler beat (Fig. 71).

Ventricular Capture (Interference Dissociation and Interference Beat)

In nodal rhythm or idioventricular rhythm with complete blockade of retrograde conduction there is atrioventricular dissociation; in such a rhythm the impulse from the S–A node may sometimes travel downwards and may prematurely discharge the A–V node or the idioventricular focus and cause a premature ventricular contraction which interferes with the existing regular rhythm; this type of premature ventricular complex arising from the forward conduction of the impulse from the S–A node is called an interference beat (ventricular capture); this type of dissociation along with the advent of such an interference beat is called the interference dissociation. In such cases the ventricular rate is usually faster than the atrial rate.

Electrocardiogram after Paroxysmal Tachycardia

After an attack of paroxysmal tachycardia has ceased, there may be ectopic beats, depression of the S–T segment and T wave inversion for hours or days in the electrocardiographic tracing.

Paced beats

Paced beats may be ventricular or atrial.

Ventricular paced beats are ventricular beats originating from artificial stimulation of the ventricular myocardium with the help of artificial pacemakers.

An artificial pacemaker is an instrument which emits electrical impulses of short duration at a desired rate so that they excite the ventricular myocardium with effective ventricular contractions at the desired rate.

An artificial pacemaker is run by a system of batteries and the ventricular myocardium is stimulated by connecting electrodes.

The pacemaker is kept outside the body in an emergency and later this is replaced by an implantable pacemaker which is embedded in the tissues of the body usually in the pectoral region of the chest.

The connecting electrodes may be applied externally (external pacemaking) over the precordium or may be fixed in the myocardium or may be introduced into the right ventricular cavity by means of an epicardial or endocardial electrodes respectively (internal pacemaking).

In the electrocardiogram the paced beats are immediately preceded by a vertical line of artificial stimulation and the QRS complexes are wide simulating left bundle-branch block; scattered P waves may be visible due to independent atrial contractions. Sometimes an impulse from the sinus node may pass through the A–V node and stimulate the ventricles when they are not in the refractory period. Thus there may be a competition between the S–A node pacemaker and the artificial pacemaker. QRS–T complexes from S–A node pacemaker are normal in duration and are regularly preceded by P waves. The paced beats may be complicated by ventricular fibrillation or other arrhythmias (Figs. 74 & 75).

Atrial paced beats are obtained from artificial stimulation of the right atrial wall in absence of A–V block. Atrial pacing is required for research and investigative purposes.

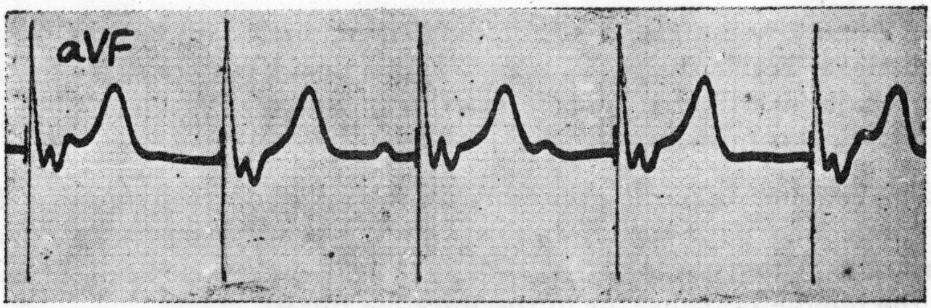

Fig. 74.

Fig. 74 shows an electrocardiogram of ventricular paced beats taken immediately after fixation of the endocardial electrode at the apex of the right ventricle; besides ventricular complexes, there are also independent regular P waves. Pacemaker 'blip' is also seen immediately before each ventricular complex.

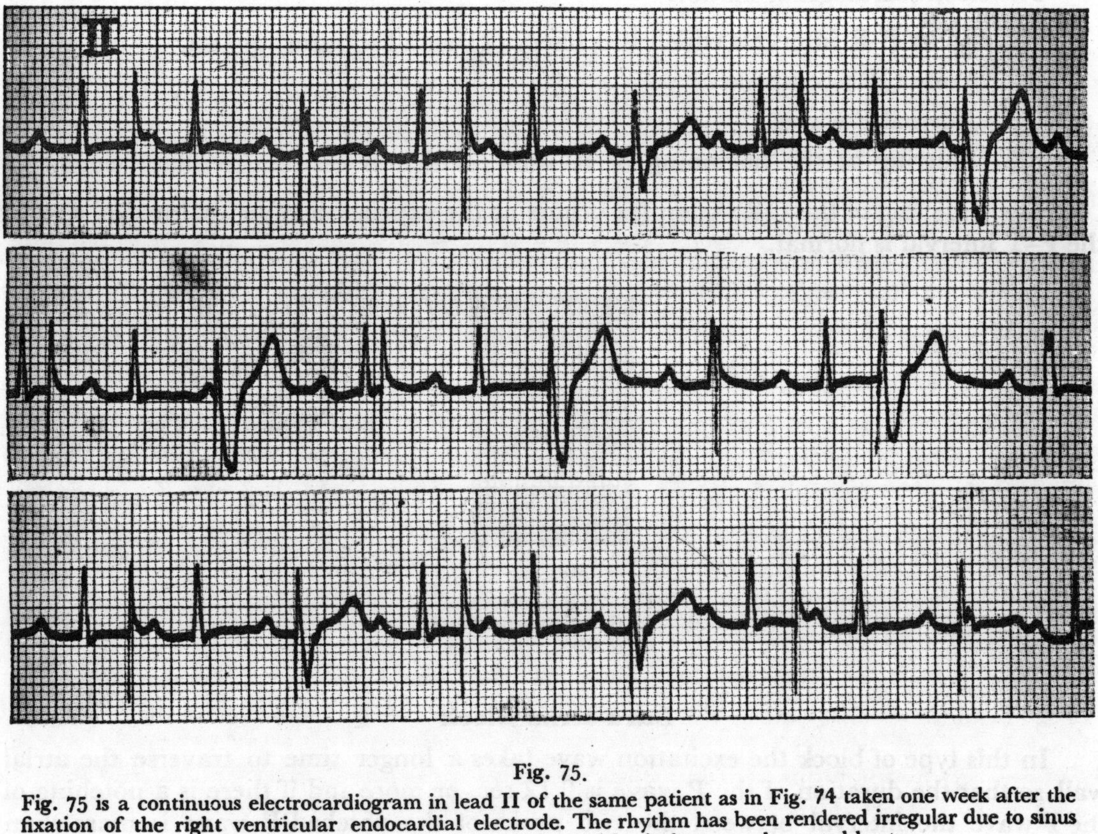

Fig. 75.

Fig. 75 is a continuous electrocardiogram in lead II of the same patient as in Fig. 74 taken one week after the fixation of the right ventricular endocardial electrode. The rhythm has been rendered irregular due to sinus node excitation also stimulating the ventricles in between the paced beats.

CHAPTER VII

CONDUCTION DEFECTS

A normal excitatory impulse is originated and conducted from the S–A node through the atrial muscle to reach the A–V node. From the A–V node the impulse travels through the bundle of His, the bundle branches, and the Purkinje fibres successively to reach the ventricular muscle.

A defective conduction of the excitatory impulse may develop due to a defect at any part of the conducting pathway; thus this may happen during the conduction of the impulse from the S–A node to the A–V node, or in the A–V node itself, or in the bundle of His, or in the bundle branches, or in the Purkinje fibres.

Wolff-Parkinson-White Syndrome (Pre-excitation Syndrome : W.P.W. Syndrome)

When there is defective conduction from the S–A node so that there is asymmetrical arrival of the impulse in the two ventricles, it is referred to as W.P.W. syndrome. In this case one ventricle is excited earlier than the other which is excited in normal time (Fig. 76).

The electrocardiogram shows:

1. Short P–R intervals which is 0·1 sec. (2½ small squares) or less.
2. Wide QRS complexes.
3. Normal P waves.
4. Slurring at the beginning of R wave, which is called the Delta wave.

The widening of the QRS complex occurs at the expense of the P–R interval so that the P–T interval is normal.

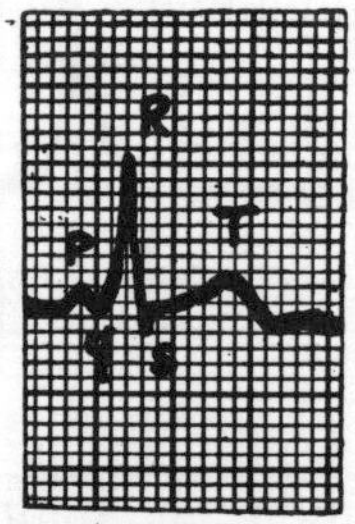

Fig. 76.

Fig. 76 is a diagrammatic representation of W.P.W. syndrome.

Intra-atrial Block

In this type of block the excitation wave takes a longer time to traverse the atrial wall so that the duration of the P wave is 0·12 sec. or more and if there is a notching of the P wave the interval between the two peaks of the notched P wave is more than 0·04 sec. This may be found in mitral valve disease, ischaemic heart disease and left ventricular hypertrophy (*vide* Review Tracing 26).

Atrio-ventricular Block

When there is defective conduction through A–V node the term heart block is used. This is classified into 4 grades or degrees:

1. 1st DEGREE HEART BLOCK

In this the P–R interval in all the leads is prolonged (more than 0·22 sec., i.e., more than 5½ small squares) without any dropping of the QRS complexes (Figs. 77, 78 & 79).

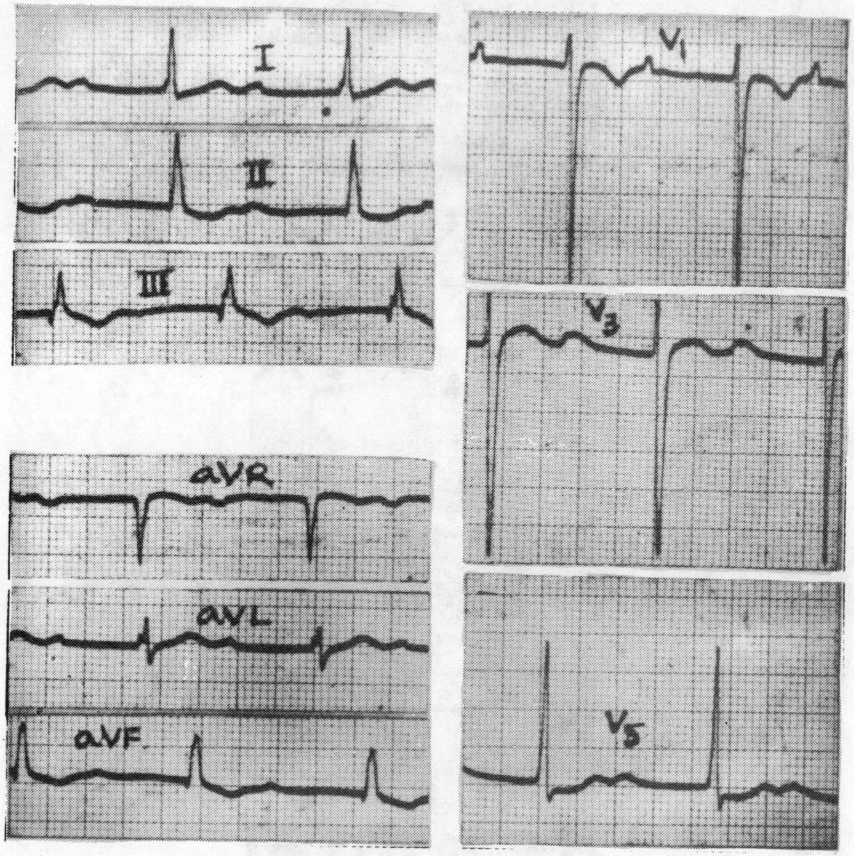

Fig. 77.

Fig. 77 shows an electrocardiogram from a case suffering from ischaemic heart disease having 1st degree heart block.

2. 2nd DEGREE HEART BLOCK

In this type there is an occasional absence of the QRS–T complex after regular P waves.

3. 3rd DEGREE HEART BLOCK

Here there is a regular dropping of the QRS–T complex after 2 or 3 or 4 or more regular P waves.

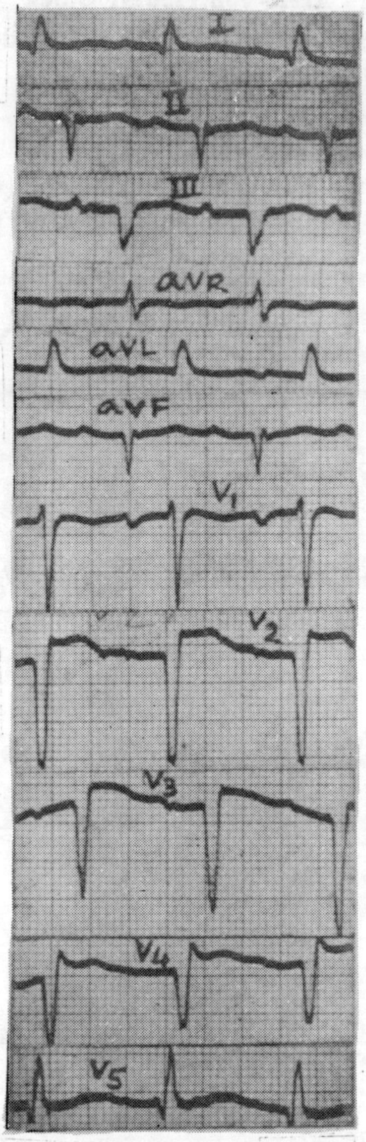

Fig. 78.

Fig. 78 is an electrocardiogram of old myocardial infarction of postero-inferior wall with acute myocardial infarction of septal wall having also 1st degree heart block.

Thus if there is one ventricular complex after two regular P waves it is called 2 : 1 A–V block, or one ventricular complex after three regular P waves it is 3 : 1 A–V block and so on. Again if there are two ventricular complexes out of three regular and successive P waves it is called 3 : 2 A–V block or three ventricular complexes out of four regular and successive P waves, it is called 4 : 3 A–V block and so on.

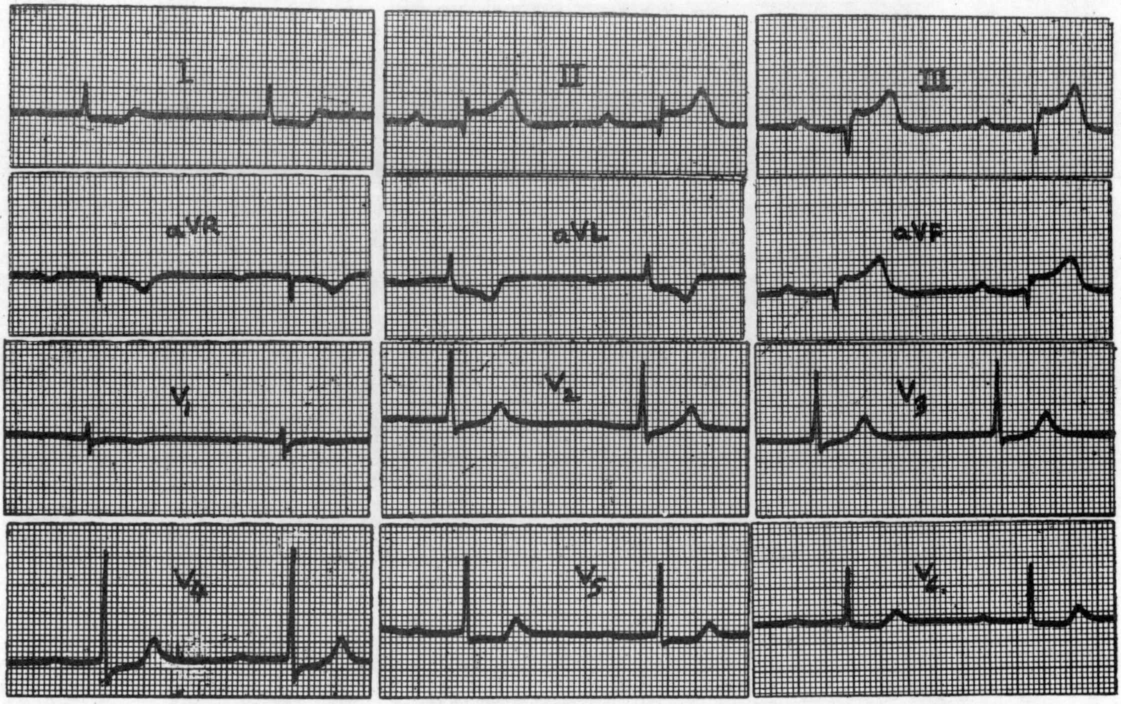

Fig. 79.

Fig. 79 is an electrocardiogram from a male patient aged 48 yrs. who had acute chest pain for the first time; the tracing was taken within 2 hours of the clinical attack; there is acute myocardial infarction of postero-inferior wall with myocardial ischaemia in the anterior wall; coving of S–T segment has not yet developed; there is sinus bradycardia and 1st degree heart block.

Wenckebach phenomenon

This is a special variety of 3rd degree A–V block where the P–R interval increases progressively in successive beats and ultimately a QRS–T complex is dropped (Type I of Mobitz). This dropping of QRS–T complex may follow a P wave after 2 or 3 or 4 or more P–QRS–T complexes (Figs. 80 & 81).

Mobitz type of heart block

This is a variety of 3rd degree heart block (Type II of Mobitz) where there is a regular dropping of QRS–T complexes following P waves after 2 or 3 or 4 or more regular P waves with ventricular complexes. In such cases P–R intervals are constant, although they may be either normal or prolonged in a particular tracing.

4. 4TH DEGREE HEART BLOCK

In this type there is complete block in the conducting pathway below the atrial level and no impulse from the sinus node can reach the ventricles.

This occurs when there is complete block at the A–V node or the bundle of His or both the bundle branches allowing no impulse to pass through them; the ventricular

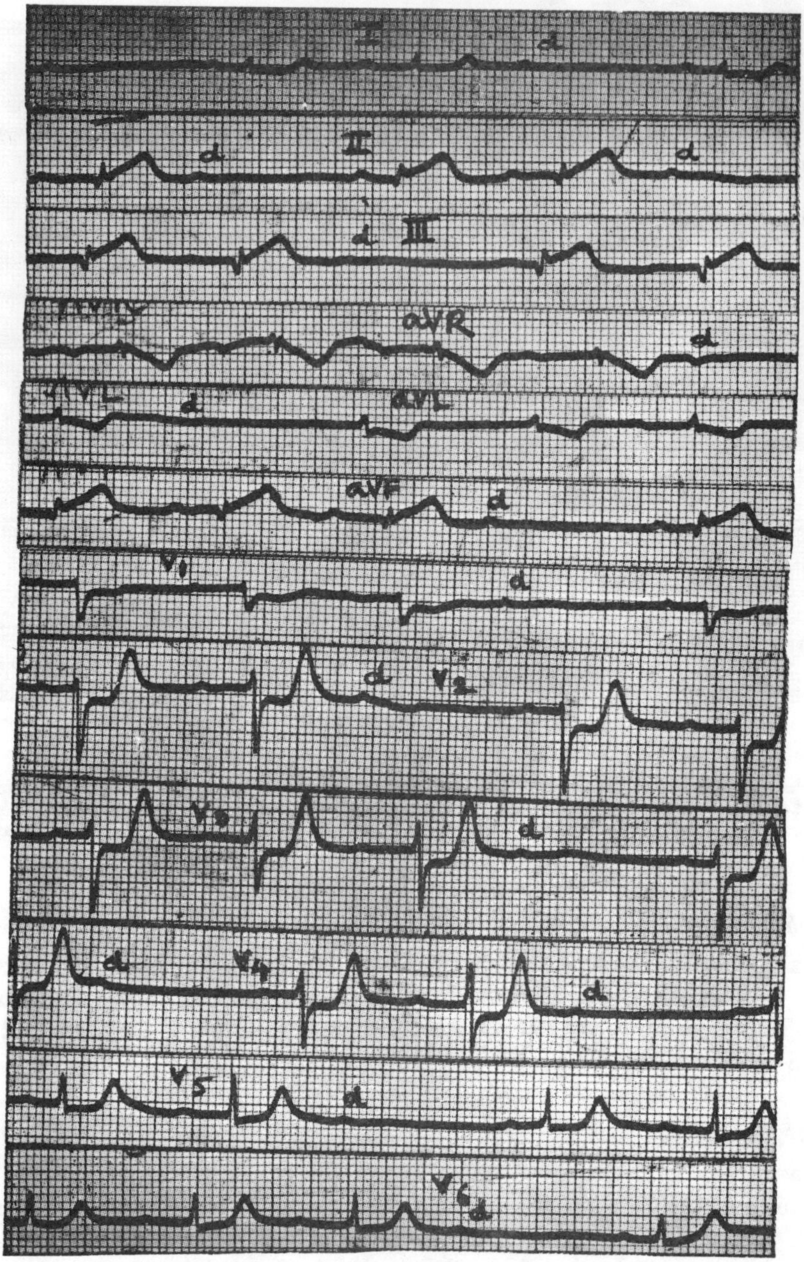

Fig. 80.

Fig. 80 shows an electrocardiographic tracing from a case of myocardial infarction having 3rd degree heart block with Wenckebach phenomenon.

excitation then takes place from an excitatory focus below the level of the block; such an excitatory focus is called an idioventricular focus and the rhythm so developed is called an idioventricular rhythm. In the electrocardiogram it is recognised by (Fig. 82):

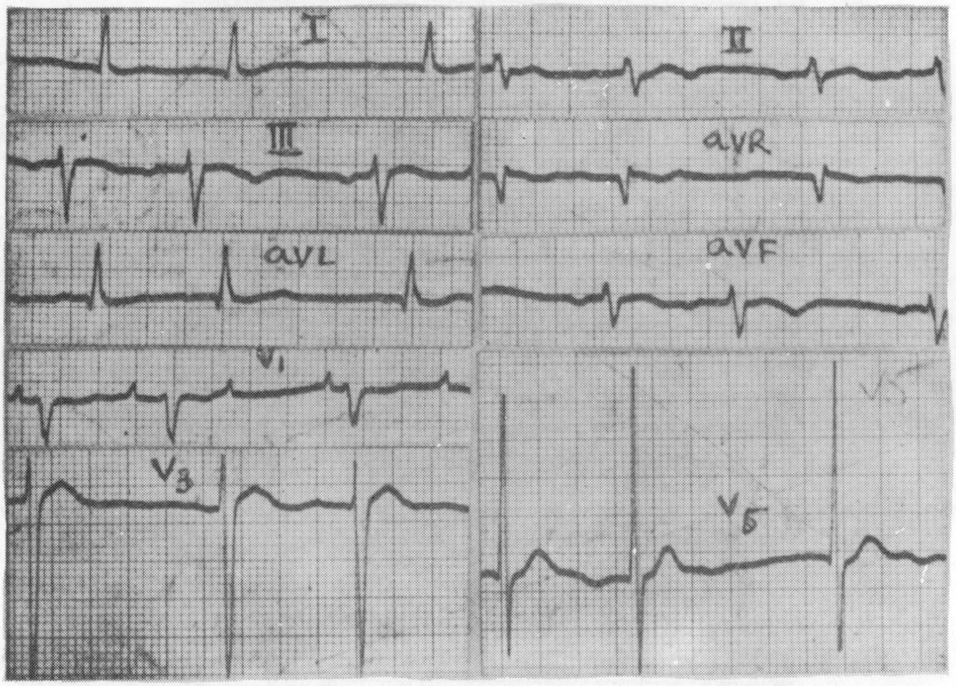

Fig. 81.

Fig. 81 is an electrocardiogram from a patient of cardiomyopathy and portal cirrhosis having Wenckebach type of heart block.

1. The P waves are at regular intervals, the atrial rate being 60 to 90/minute.
2. Slow ventricular rate which is usually below 40/minute (usually 36/minute).
3. Similar QRS complexes in a particular lead and these complexes are usually widened.

When the ventricular rate is higher than the atrial rate the term A–V dissociation is used.

Sometimes the duration of the QRS complexes may not be increased. In such cases the excitable focus is situated in the bundle of His itself.

In congenital complete heart block the ventricular rate is high and may be influenced by exertion, emotion and drugs.

Bundle-Branch Block (B.B.B.)

In this case there is a block in one bundle branch or in both the bundle branches being involved alternately. When there is a complete block in both the bundle branches simultaneously, the defect will behave like complete heart block. When there is a block in one of the bundle branches it may involve either the right or the left bundle branch or both the bundle branches singly and alternately.

In B.B.B. a P wave precedes the QRS complex, and the direction of the T wave is opposite to that of the main deflection of the QRS complex.

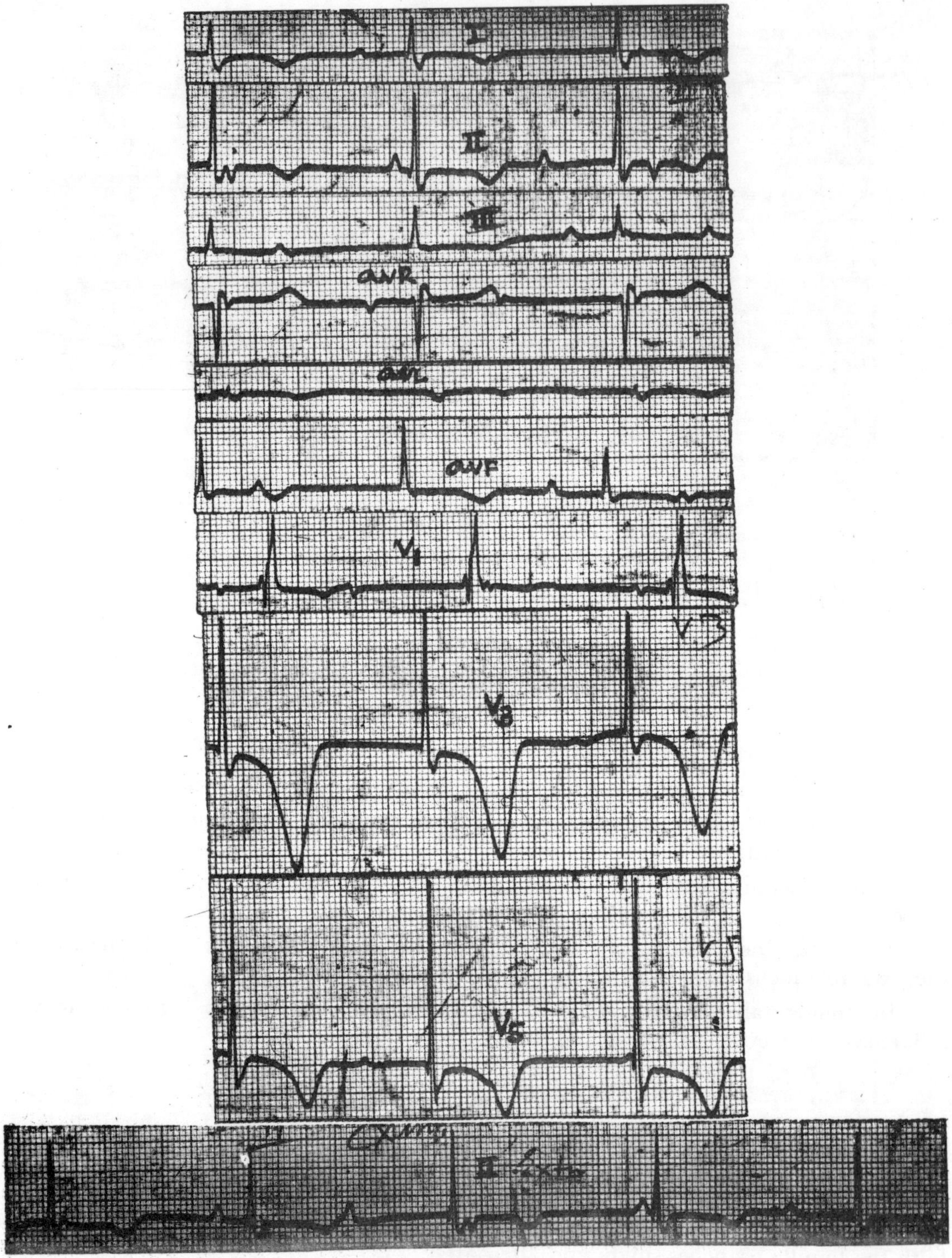

Fig. 82.

Fig. 82 is an electrocardiogram showing complete heart block, left ventricular hypertrophy and ischaemic heart disease.

A. RIGHT BUNDLE-BRANCH BLOCK (R.B.B.B.)

This may be diagnosed from the following features (Fig. 83):

1. The intrinsicoid deflection in lead V_1 is more than 0·02 sec. (i.e., more than ½ small square).
2. The QRS complexes in lead V_1 show the rSR′ pattern, i.e., a small upward deflection, (r wave) and then a downward deflection (S wave) and then another upward deflection. (R′ wave).
3. The S wave in lead I is slurred.

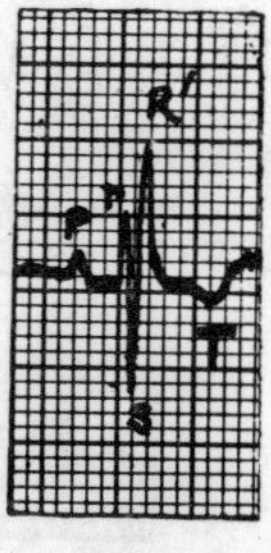

Fig. 83.

Fig. 83 is a diagrammatic representation of right bundle-branch block (complete).

B. LEFT BUNDLE-BRANCH BLOCK (L.B.B.B.)

This may be diagnosed from the following features (Figs. 84 & 85):

1. The Intrinsicoid deflection in lead V_5 is more than 0·04 sec. (i.e., more than one small square).
2. The QRS complexes in leads I and V_5 show a slurred or notched R wave (the so-called M or W pattern).

If the duration of the QRS complex in the standard leads in bundle-branch block is less than 0·12 sec., i.e., less than 3 small squares, the B.B.B. is incomplete; if the duration of the QRS complex in standard leads is 0·12 sec. the B.B.B. is complete.

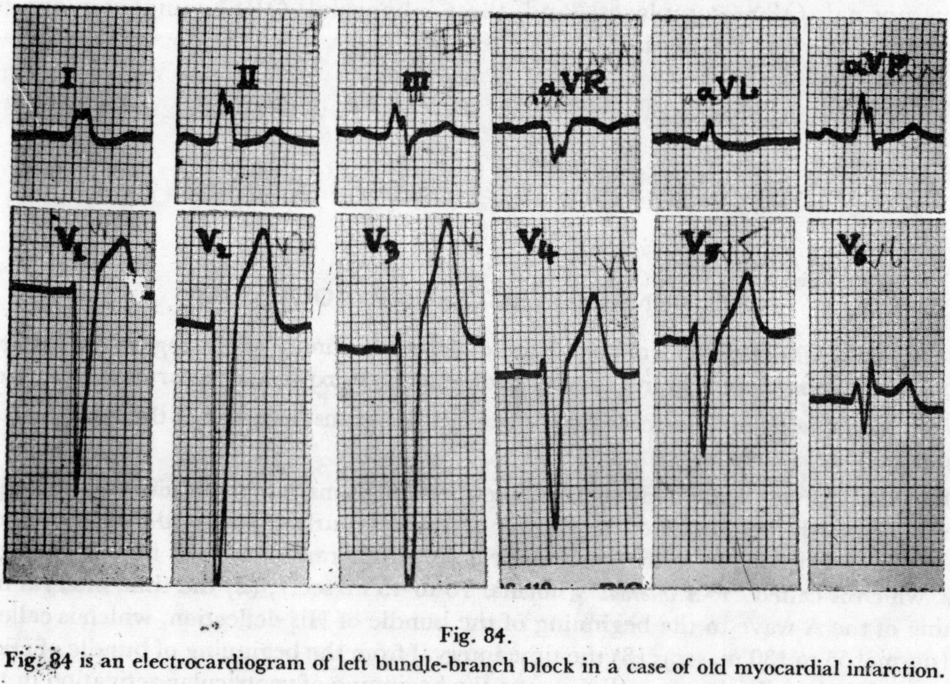

Fig. 84.

Fig. 84 is an electrocardiogram of left bundle-branch block in a case of old myocardial infarction.

Arborisation Block (Intraventricular Conduction Defect)

In this type of block there is usually widening of the QRS complex to more than

0·12 sec. in the standard leads and the QRS complex does not show definite pattern of either R.B.B.B. or L.B.B.B.

In arborisation block normal P waves precede the widened QRS complexes.

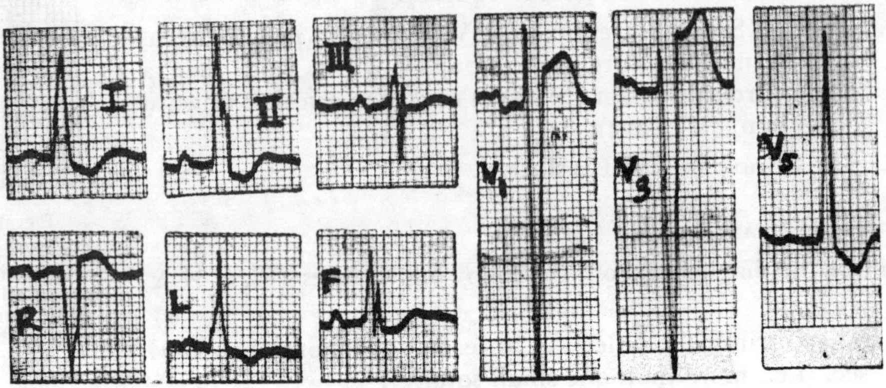

Fig. 85.

Fig. 85 is an electrocardiogram of left bundle-branch block.

Aberrant Ventricular Conduction (Ventricular Aberration)

In this type of abnormal conduction the electrocardiogram shows a B.B.B. pattern or arborisation block pattern (commonly R.B.B.B.) of one or more QRS complexes in between normal QRS complexes, and these abnormal QRS complexes are usually preceded by abnormal P waves.

HIS BUNDLE ELECTROCARDIOGRAPHY

Electrocardiograms taken from this site i.e. from the bundle of His region are not available routinely as the procedure requires special knowledge and experience apart from the gadgets.

With the bundle of His recordings electrocardiograms from one of the body surface leads are simultaneously taken.

The P-R interval of the body surface electrocardiograms may be divided into 3 segments: (1) the time from the beginning of the P wave of the body surface lead to the beginning of the A wave i.e. the first deflection in the low atrial electrocardiogram of the His bundle electrocardiography, which is called "*P-A interval*" (normal 10 to 45 m. sec.); (2) the time interval from the beginning of the A wave to the beginning of the bundle of His deflection, which is called "A-H time" (normal 55 to 130 m. sec); (3) the time interval from the beginning of bundle of His deflection in the His bundle electrocardiogram to the beginning of ventricular activation in the electrocardiogram of the body surface lead which is called the "H-V interval" (normal 30 to 55 m sec.). (See fig 86)

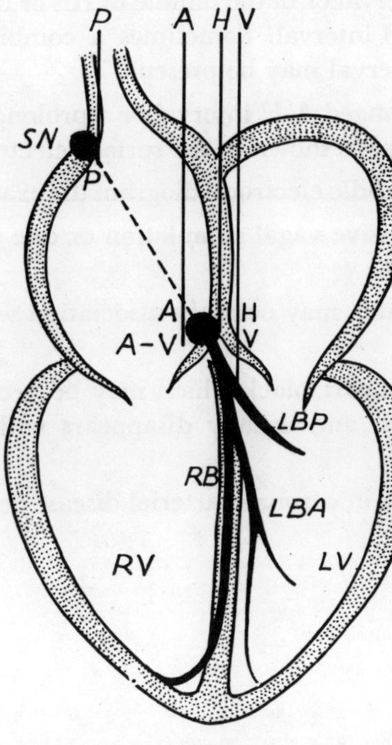

Fig. 86 Schematic representation of time intervals of different segments of His bundle electrocardiography.

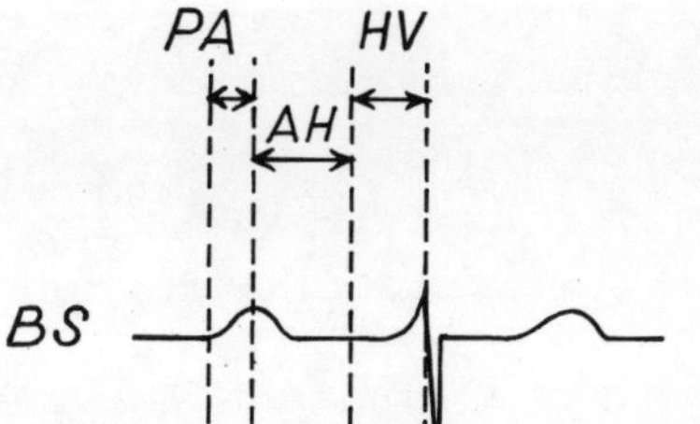

Fig. 87 Schematic illustration of body surface electrocardiogram (BS) and His bundle electrocardiogram showing P-A time interval (PA), A-H time interval (AH) and H-V time interval (HV). A=atrial depolarisation, H=His bundle depolarisation, V=depolarisation of upper ventricular septum

The P-A interval is, however, of little clinical significance and represents intra-atrial conduction time (upper to lower atrium); A-H interval represents A-V nodal conduction time; H-V interval represents His-Purkinje conduction time.

When there is a first-degree A-V block recognised by a prolonged P-R interval, the block may be situated either above the bundle of His i.e. in the A-V node which gives a prolonged A-H interval with a normal H-V interval or in the bundle of His or below it giving rise to a prolonged H-V interval with a normal A-H interval. Sometimes a combination of both prolonged A-H interval and prolonged H-V interval may be present.

In some cases either a prolonged A-H interval or a prolonged H-V interval may be present along with a normal P-R interval as shown in the surface electrocardiogram.

Thus with the help of His bundle electrocardiogram the exact site of block may be detected.

The A-V block due to excessive vagal stimulation or due to digitalis toxicity may be easily controlled, if carefully examined.

First degree heart block which may occur in association with acute infectious diseases, is a reversible lesion.

The first or second degree heart block which may be present in acute rheumatic fever, indicates rheumatic myocarditis, and usually disappears with the subsidence of rheumatic fever.

The prognosis of heart block in coronary arterial disease depends on the severity of the coronary disease.

CHAPTER VIII

SICK SINUS SYNDROME

Definition : Sick Sinus Syndrome is a form of cardiac arrhythmia arising out of subnormal function of the sino-atrial node so that an unusual delay occurs to build up its charge to a firing level due to loss of pacemaking cells of S-A node. The patient often complaints of vertigo, syncope and a sense of discomfort in the chest (Fig. 88).

Disease of the artio-ventricular node may be associated with it and a careful search should always be made for any evidence of such associated involvement.

Types of presentation

1. Sinus bradycardia :

The subject develops an excessively slow heart rate with a sinus rhythm which does not respond adequately to physical exercise.

2. Sinoatrial 'exit block':

In this type the tissues immediately around the S-A node develop a 'block' so that the impulses from the S-A node cannot traverse the refractory tissue around the S-A node easily and reach the atrial tissues. In the electrocardiogram there are prolonged pauses irregularly and recurrently following regular sinus beats.

3. Classical type of sino-atrial block :

In this classical type of S-A block there is usually 2 : 1 block intermittently so that the interval between the two S-A beats become exactly double or multiple thereof the interval between the two regular sinus beats.

4. Long post-ectopic pauses :

When the S-A node is sick and sluggish it will require a longer time to rebuild its charge to a firing level after being discharged by an ectopic beat and thus the post-ectopic pause will be unusually prolonged. The prolonged post-ectopic pause is often followed by an escape ectopic beat.

5. Bradycardia-tachycardia syndrome :

In this type of arrhythmia a slow sinus rate is often followed by frequent pauses and is interrupted by recurrent paroxysms of atrial flutter, atrial fibrillation, a combination of both atrial flutter and fibrillation or supraventricular tachycardia.

Diagnosis

When there is a history of recurrent episodes of syncope or vertigo existence of sick sinus syndrome should be considered.

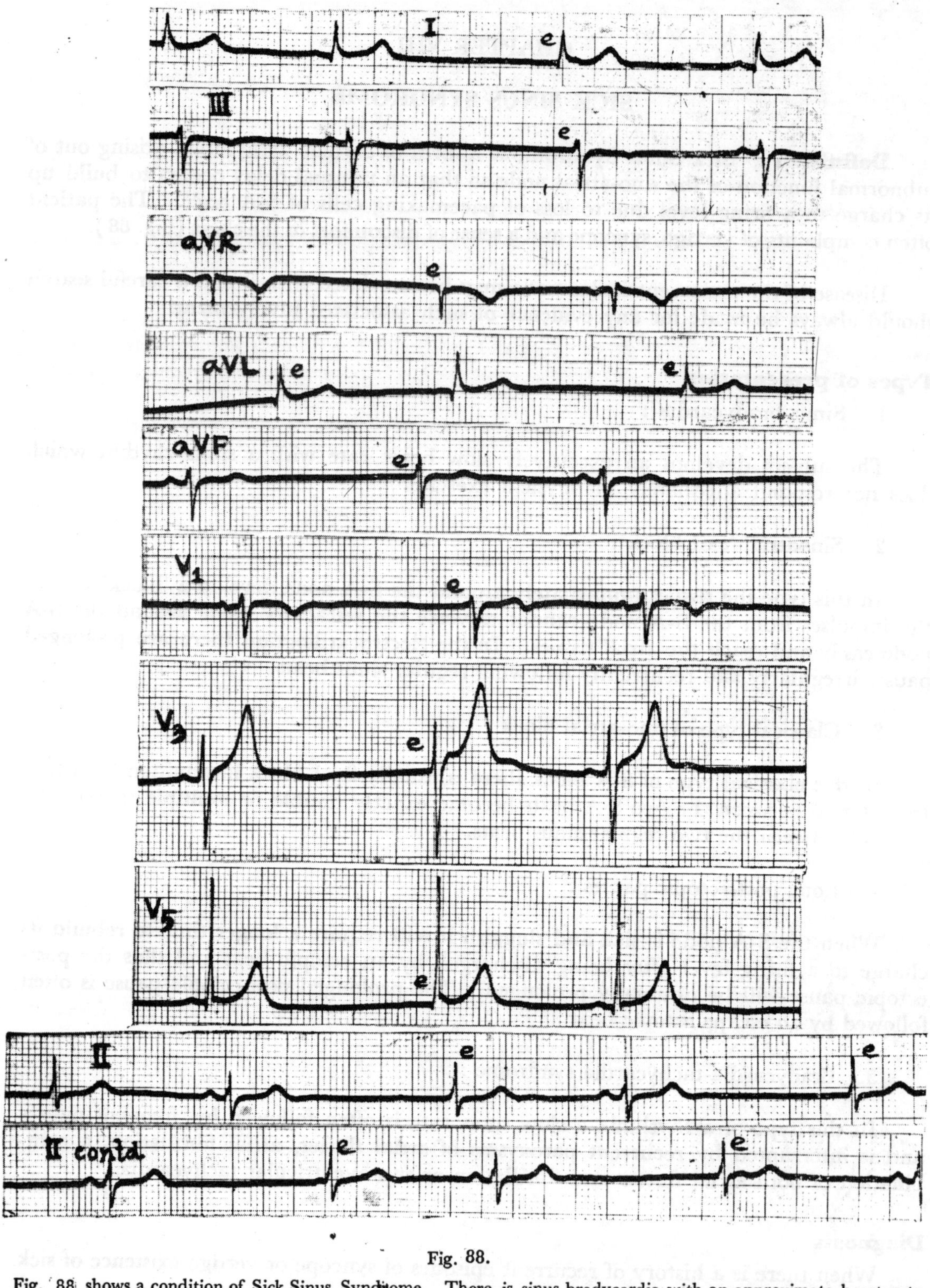

Fig. 88.

Fig. 88 shows a condition of Sick Sinus Syndrome. There is sinus bradycardia with an approximate heart rate of about 46/minute. The Sinus Node is very sluggish and is often intervened by a nodal escape

Electrocardiographic manifestations of sick sinus syndrome as explained above should establish the diagnosis.

When the electrocardiograms supplied are not helpful a continuous cardiac monitoring of such patients for 12 to 24 hours may help to exhibit the cardiac irregularities as stated above and confirm the diagnosis of sick sinus syndrome. A Holter monitor recording is most suitable for this purpose. Such cardiac irregularities can, however, be correlated with the symptoms of the patients.

An intravenous injection of atropine sulphate 1 mg. increases the pulse rate by 50% or more in a normal person. A person with sick sinus syndrome may not respond or may respond with an increase of heart rate by 25% or less after the atropine injection.

A slow recovery time of the sluggish S-A node following its premature discharge by an ectopic beat may be brought out by what is called 'overdrive suppression' of S-A node. In this procedure an atrial pacing is done at a rate of 150 per minute for 30 seconds and then the pacing is stopped. In a person with a normal S-A node the time from the end of atrial pacing to the appearance of first heart beat is about 1½ seconds. A person with a sick sinus syndrome the above pause is 3 seconds or more.

With the atrial pacer in position but turned off, a carotid sinus stimulation test may be done by gentle massaging of the carotid sinus on one side. Some patients of sick sinus syndrome may show long pauses after this mechanical stimulation of the carotid sinus. In case of an unusually long pause the atrial pacing may be started.

CHAPTER IX

FASCICULAR BLOCK

The bundle branch system in the ventricles of the heart consists of right bundle branch, left and right divisions of the left bundle branch. These three divisions of the bundle of His are the three fascicles of the bundle branch system.

A block in the bundle branch system may involve any one or two or all the three fascicles when it is described as monofascicular, bifascicular and trifascicular block respectively.

A block in the bundle branch system is not influenced by antivagal drugs or by digitalis. Unlike complete heart block at A-V node Stokes-Adams fits are common after complete block in bundle branch system.

Disease or dysfunction of the bundle branch system may cause delayed conduction, intermittent conduction or complete failure of conduction of the impulses from above and may give rise to all degrees of heart block.

Monofascicular block

The left bundle branch arising from the distal end of the bundle of His divides into an anterior fascicle and a posterior fascicle. When one of these fascicles is blocked ventricular excitation occurs through the other functioning fascicle.

When there is an isolated transmission of the impulse through the posterior fascicle, anterior fascicle being blocked (left anterior fascicular block), there is an extreme left axis deviation (−45 degrees or more), the QRS being 0·11 sec., lead I showing a qR pattern and lead III showing an rS pattern.

When there is an isolated transmission of the impulse through the anterior fascicle only, the posterior fascicle being blocked (left posterior fascicular block), there is an extreme right axis deviation (+120 degrees or more).

Thus the left anterior fascicular block or left anterior hemiblock is diagnosed by extreme left axis deviation (−45 degrees or greater), slightly widened QRS complexes (0·11 second) and a qR configuration in lead I with an rS configuration in lead III.

The left posterior fascicular block or left posterior hemiblock is recognised by extreme right axis deviation (+120 degrees or greater), slightly widened QRS complexes (0·11 sec) and an rS configuration in lead I with a qR configuration in lead III, provided other causes of extreme right axis deviation have been excluded (Fig. 89).

Bifascicular block

When there is complete right bundle branch block associated with a block of any one of the two fascicles of the left bundle branch, the term 'bifascicular block' is used.

Occurrence of a right bundle branch block with an extreme left or an extreme right axis deviation gives a clue to the diagnosis of bifascicular block (Fig. 90).

Trifascicular block

If there is a delay in the atrio-ventricular conduction time along with bifascicular block as mentioned above, the delay is likely to be due to a fault in the remaining functioning fascicle and such a type of heart block is called a trifascicular block.

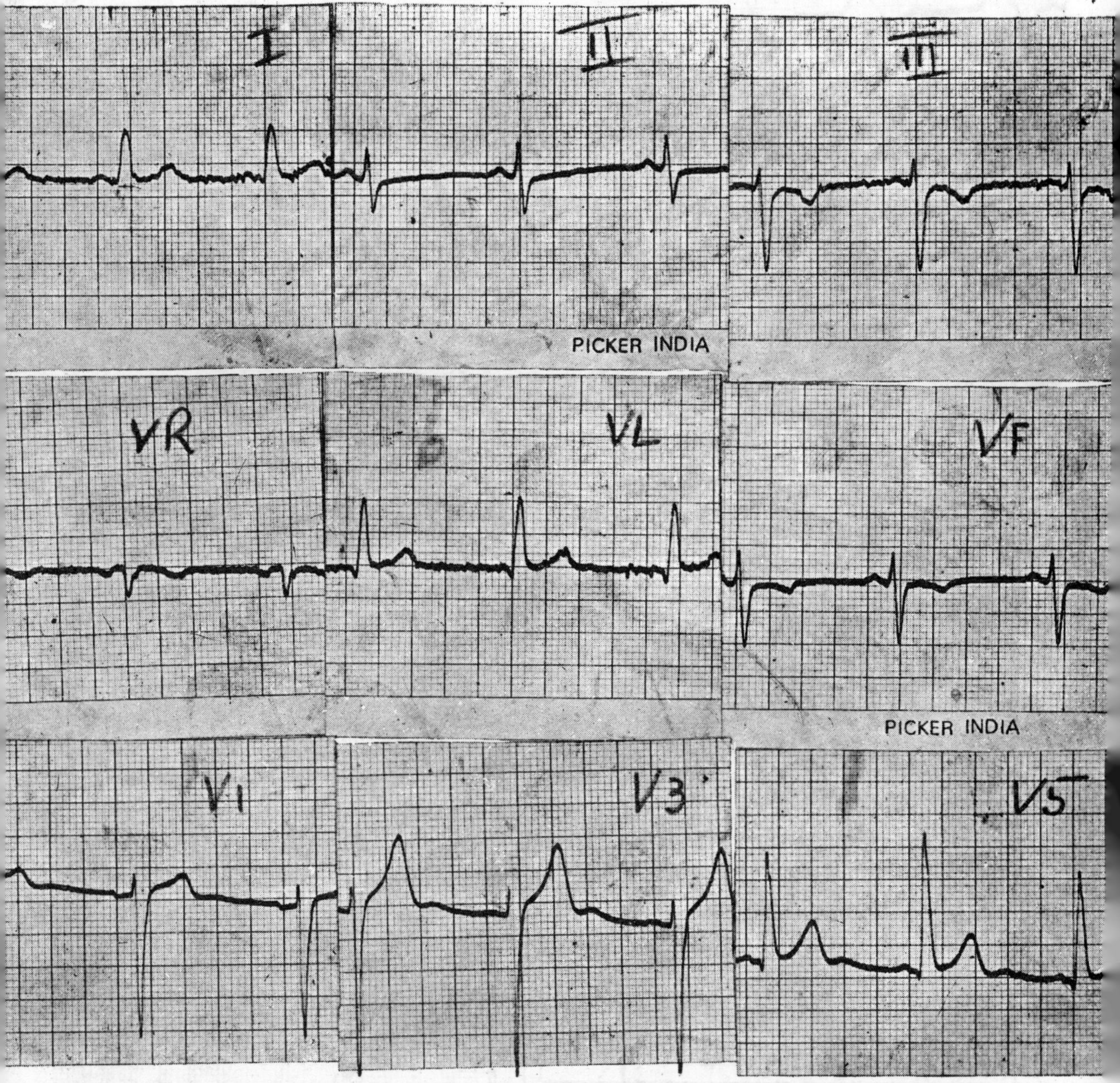

Fig. 89

Fig. 89 shows a monofascicular block; there is left anterior hemiblock recognised by a gross left axis deviation, QRS duration of 0 11 sec; there is also left ventricular hypertrophy and ischaemic myocardial changes of postero-inferior wall.

Thus the trifascicular block is diagnosed by the presence of a first degree or second degree heart block along with a bifascicular block. Such a condition is likely to be followed by complete heart block sooner or later and is described as a complete trifascicular block. However a complete A-V nodal block along with widened QRS complexes may originate from A-V nodal block along with a bundle branch block (Fig. 91)

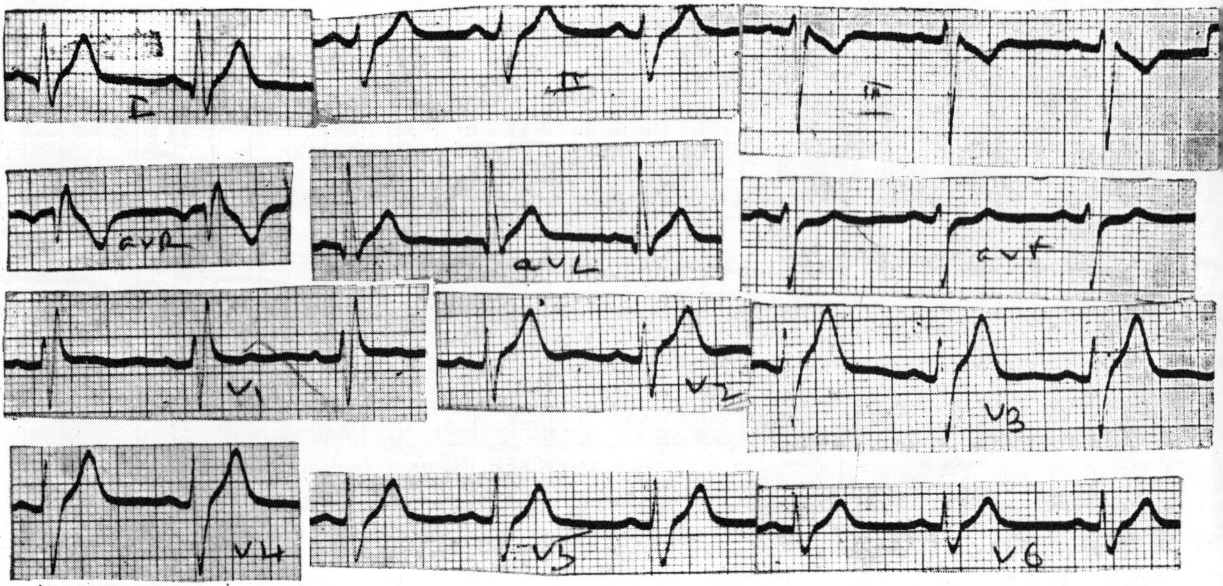

Fig. 90.

Fig. 90. shows bifascicular block; there is complete right bundle branch block along with left anterior hemi-block.

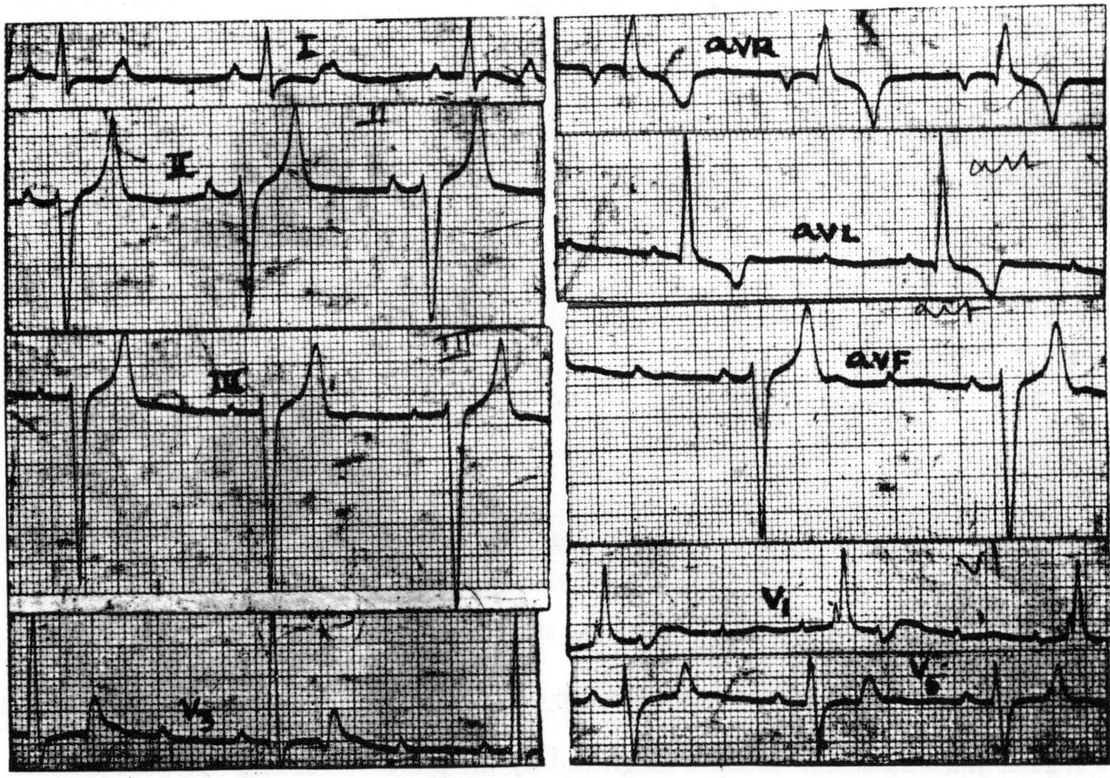

Fig. 91.

Fig. 91 shows gross left axis deviation, gross left ventricular hypertrophy and complete right bundle branch block with irregular dropping of ventricular beats (2 : 1, 3 : 1 block, etc.); presence of left anterior hemiblock with right bundle branch block constitute bifascicular block; association of these with irregular dropping of ventricular complexes indicate trifascicular block.

CHAPTER IX(A)

CARDIAC PACING AND ELECTROCARDIOGRAM

Electrostimulation was first attempted on dead animals or humans with a view to revive them in the 18th century. In 1952, Zoll successfully employed electrostimulation of heart in a case of Adams-Stokes syndrome. In the following decade the basic methods of cardiac pacing had been established. Initially, intermittent myocardial stimulations were effected with the help of an external pulse generator. In 1960, Elmquist and Senning advocated the use of an implantable pacemaker where the battery could be recharged externally requiring external appliances. Subsequently, pulse generators powered by mercury-zinc batteries were introduced.

Initially, the pacing by the artificial pacemaker was asynchronous and the pacemaker had a fixed rate ignoring the nature of the existing cardiac rhythm; this type of fixed rate pacemaker beat introduces the possibility of competition with the spontaneous beat from the natural pacemaker of the heart. Subsequently, various types of greatly improved pacemakers came into the market such as atrial pacing, ventricular pacing, atrio-ventricular pacing—all without sensing and without synchronicity. Later, atrial pacing and atrial sensing (triggered mode), ventricular pacing and ventricular sensing (triggered mode and ventricular synchronous), ventricular pacing and atrial sensing (triggered mode and atrial synchronous) had been developed. Still later, atrial pacing and atrial sensing (inhibited mode), ventricular pacing and ventricular sensing (ventricular inhibited) atrioventricular pacing and ventricular sensing, inhibited mode (A-V sequential demand) were developed.

The pattern of ECG tracings would depend on the site of placement of the pacemaker lead in the myocardium.

An unipolar pacemaker records large pacemaker spikes in the ECG tracing. A tripolar pacemaker gives rise to small spikes in the ECG tracing.

There are three modes of cardiac pacing :

(i) External pacing is used in an emergency which is painful to a conscious patient.

(ii) Internal pacing where the power source is situated outside the body of the patient. This is accomplished by inserting the electrode into the myocardium through an arm vein or nerve vein or by direct puncture of myocardial tissue through the chest wall. This is also followed in an emergency.

(iii) Internal pacing with the power generator implanted into the body of the patient; in this situation myocardial stimulation is effected through a catheter electrode placed in the myocardium of the left ventricle by thoracotomy (left ventricular epicardial pacemaker) or through a cathode electrode planted in the endocardium of the apex of the right ventricle through an arm vein or nerve vein (right ventricular endocardial pacemaker).

The power unit is placed in the abdominal wall or in the axillary or pectoral region of the chest well. The power unit then operates through a catheter lead being embedded in the myocardium either through the endocardium (endocardial lead) or through the epicardium (epicardial lead). The pattern of ECG tracing varies according to the position of the placement of the catheter lead, and the type of the pacemaker used.

In the following pages patterns of ECG tracings in different types of artificial pacemakers of the insertions are shown.

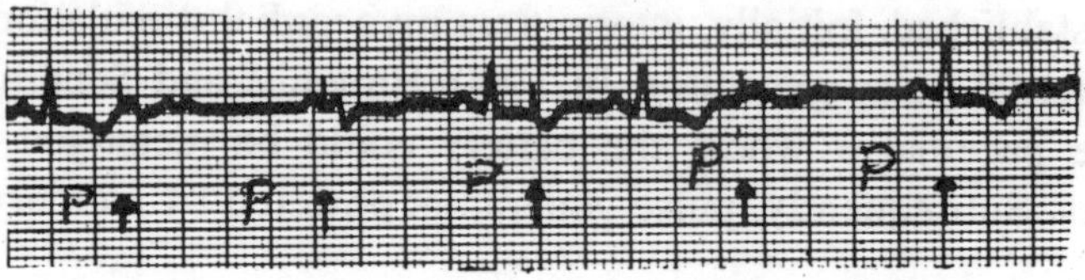

Fig. A_1 : The above ECG tracing is from a patient with a tripolar left ventricular epicardial asynchronous (fixed rate) pacemaker; the artificial pacemaker (P) discharges regularly at a rate of 65/min. The ventricle responds to the normal sino-atrial node or to the artificial pacemaker.

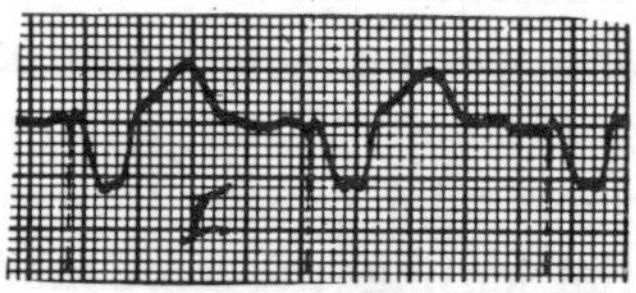

Fig. A_2 : The above ECG tracing is that of a patient having unipolar left ventricular epicardial pacemaker giving rise to large pace spikes.

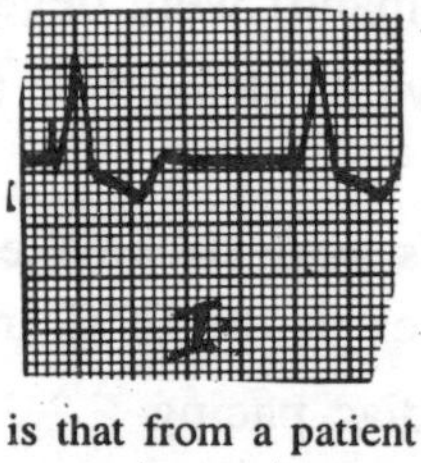

Fig A_3 : The above ECG tracing is that from a patient with a tripolar right ventricular endocardial pacemaker situated in the right ventricular apex.

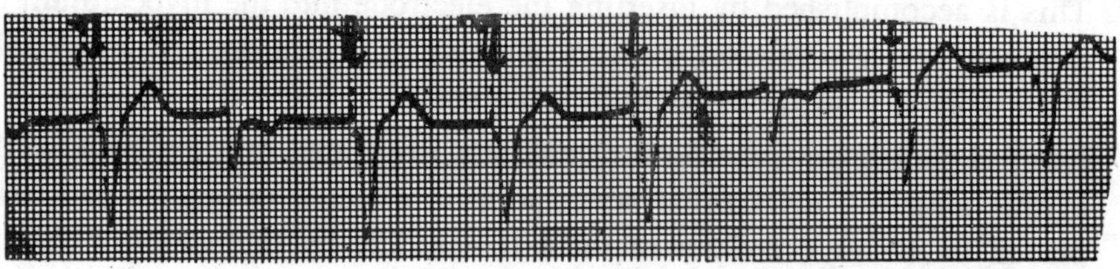

Fig. A_4 : The above ECG tracing is that from a patient with a ventricular demand pacemaker. The artificial pacemaker activity is indicated by an arrow. There is no competition between natural (spontaneous) and artificial pacemaker activities.

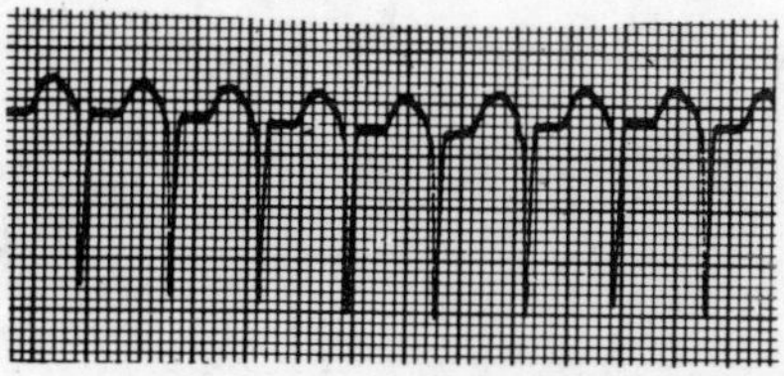

(i)

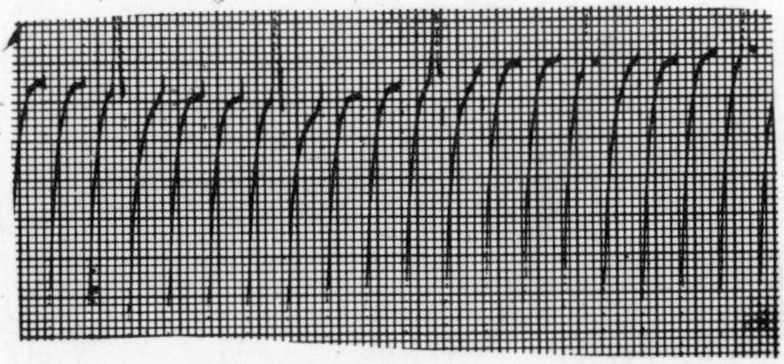

(ii)

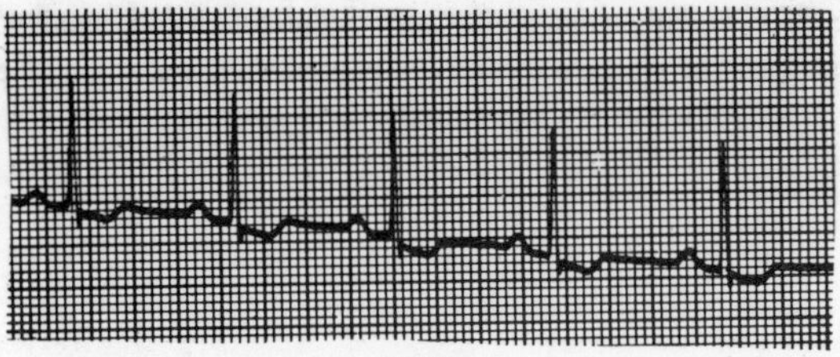

(iii)

Fig. A_5 : This is an ECG tracing from a case of paroxysmal atrial tachycardia (i). Right atrial pacing was done by an implanted artificial pacemaker. The right atrium was stimulated at a rate higher than that of atrial rate of paroxysmal atrial tachycardia (ii). This interrupted the re-entry pathway which resulted in the reversion to sinus rhythm (iii).

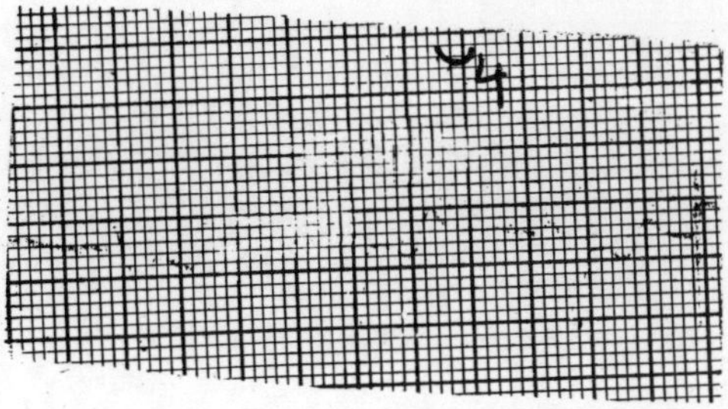

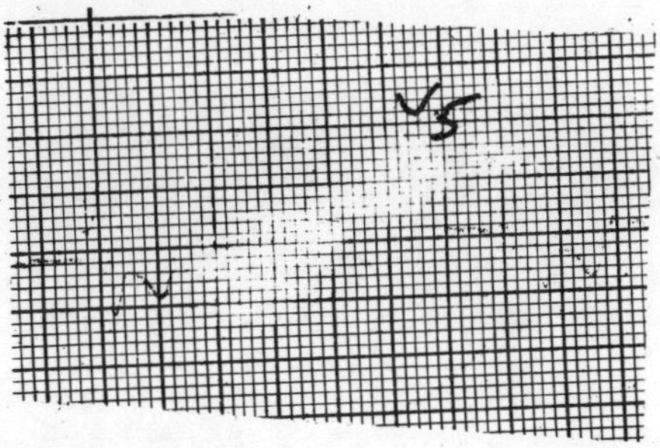

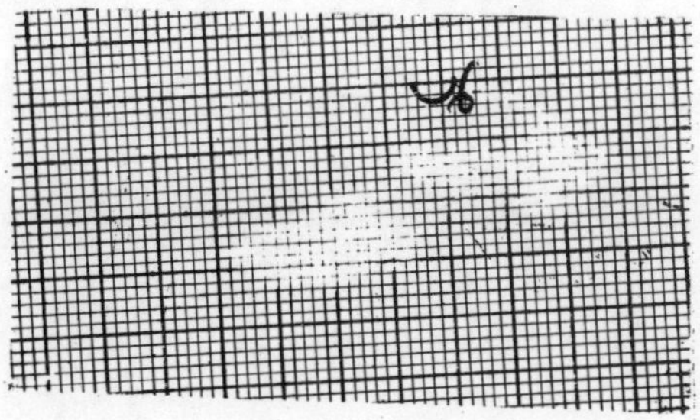

Fig. A_6 : The above ECG tracing was taken from a male patient, aged 83 years, with ischemic heart disease having an artificial pacemaker with an unipolar endocardial lead fixed at the apex of the right ventricle.

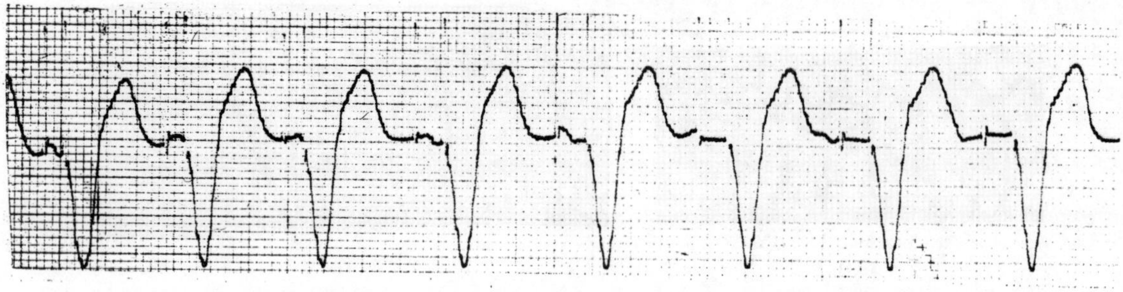

Fig. A_7 : The above ECG tracing was taken from a patient, male, aged 65 years, with a A-V sequential pacemaker; the pacemaker spikes precede each atrial and each ventricular depolarisations sequentially one after the other.

CHAPTER X

RHEUMATIC HEART DISEASE

Rheumatic Fever

The electrocardiogram may show temporarily 1st degree heart block, i.e., prolongation of the P–R interval without any other abnormality (about 30% of the cases); 2nd and 3rd degree heart block are rare; complete heart block is exceptional; the heart block is usually reversible and may be abolished temporarily by intravenous injection of 1–2 mgm. of atropine sulphate; rarely the heart block may be permanent.

The electrocardiogram may show elevated S–T segment with flattened or inverted T wave due to accompanying rheumatic pericarditis in about 10% of the cases.

Consequences of valve disease during acute rheumatic fever such as aortic incompetence, and mitral incompetence, may be shown in the electrocardiographic tracing. There may be different types of cardiac arrhythmias.

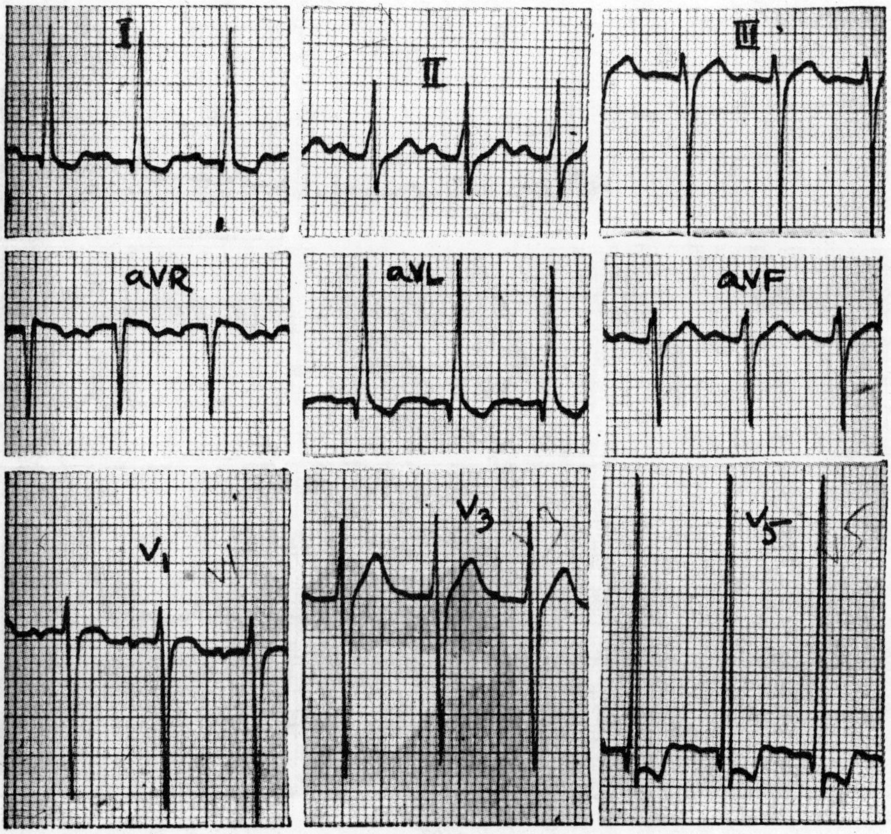

Fig. 92.

Fig. 92 is an electrocardiographic tracing from a case of gross mitral incompetence with congestive cardiac failure; the patient was digitalised; there is a gross left ventricular hypertrophy and dilatation and digitalis effect.

Mitral Incompetence

Left ventricular dominance may be present in the electrocardiographic tracing, i.e., a tall R wave, a small Q wave, and a prominent pointed T wave in the left ventricular surface leads (Review Tracing 11); S–T segment depression and T wave inversion are present over the left ventricle when there is marked left ventricular dilatation (Fig. 92). If there is an increase in the pulmonary vascular resistance there may be right ventricular dominance. P mitrale may be present. There may be different types of cardiac arrhythmias and very rarely heart block.

Mitral Stenosis

The electrocardiogram may be normal in mild cases. In others the P wave may be wide (i.e., more than 0·1 sec.) and bifid. If the P wave is tall (more than 2·5 mm. in height) it indicates increased pulmonary vascular resistance or tricuspid valve disease or right-sided congestive cardiac failure. Evidence of right ventricular preponderance (tall R wave in V_1) with or without marked clockwise rotation indicates pulmonary arterial hypertension. Cardiac arrhythmias such as atrial fibrillation, atrial flutter, etc., and exceptionally different types of heart block may be present (Fig. 93).

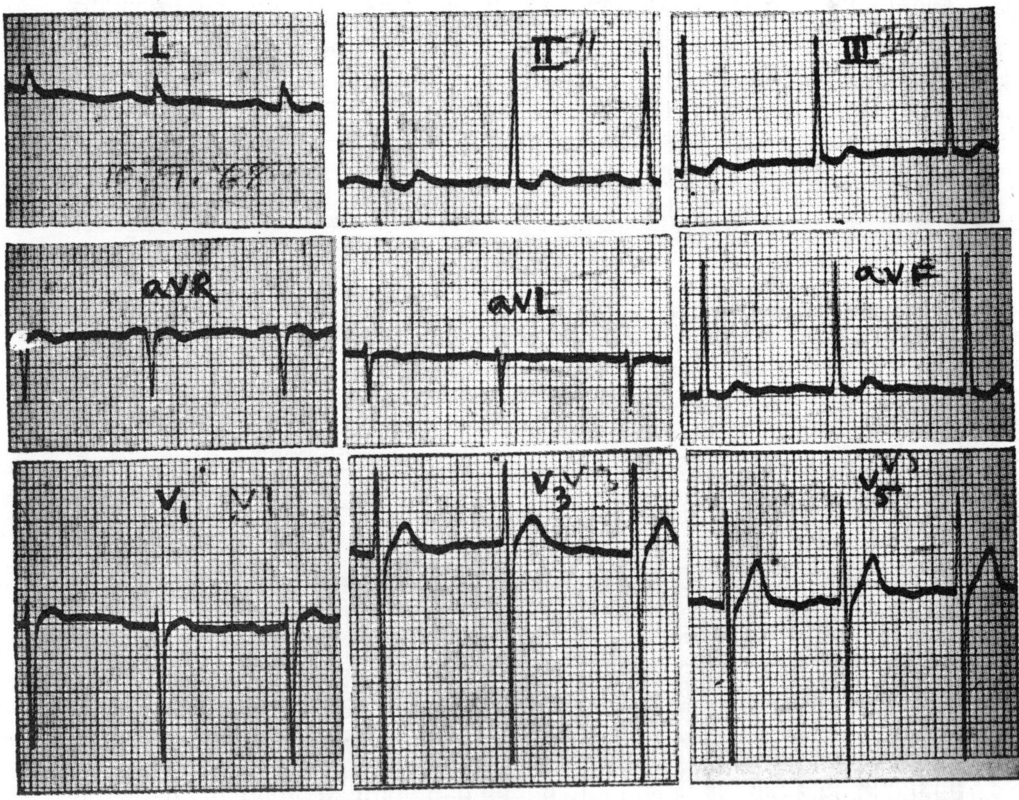

Fig. 93.

Fig. 93 is an electrocardiogram from a case of mitral stenosis showing left atrial enlargement.

There may be evidence of coronary insufficiency (depression of the S–T segment) in some cases of tight mitral stenosis.

If the electrocardiogram shows associated left ventricular enlargement, involvement of the aortic valve, hypertension, associated mitral incompetence, thyrotoxicosis, anaemia, etc., should be considered.

Aortic Incompetence

The electrocardiogram may be normal or may show evidence of left ventricular hypertrophy with or without asymmetrical inversion of the T wave in left ventricular surface leads depending on the presence or absence of the left ventricular dilatation respectively (Fig. 94). There may be S–T segment depression in case of gross aortic incompetence especially in syphilitic variety. Cardiac arrhythmias such as atrial fibrillation, paroxysmal tachycardias, etc., and heart block of different degrees may be present.

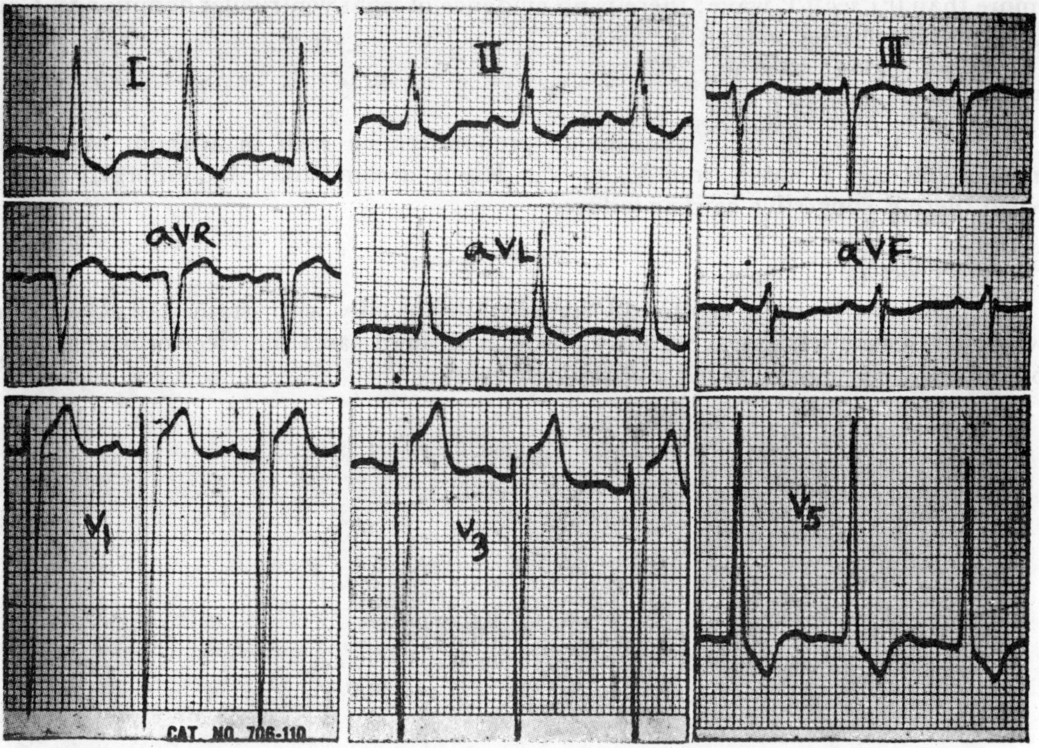

Fig. 94.

Fig. 94 is an electrocardiogram of a patient who had mitral stenosis, mitral incompetence, aortic stenosis and aortic incompetence; the tracing shows gross left ventricular hypertrophy and left atrial enlargement.

Aortic Stenosis

The electrocardiogram usually shows a vertical lie due to concentric hypertrophy of the left ventricle without dilatation.

A very high voltage of R wave is seen in V_5 and V_6.

In all the three standard leads there may be prominent R waves without any S waves; when the left ventricular hypertrophy is associated with such a pattern it is called concordant type of left ventricular hypertrophy; there is usually a depression of S–T segment and an asymmetrical inversion of the T wave in left ventricular surface leads.

There may be left bundle-branch block and A–V nodal block of various degrees in some cases.

Cardiac arrhythmias such as atrial fibrillation, paroxysmal tachycardias, etc., may occur.

Tricuspid Incompetence

In the electrocardiographic tracing there is right ventricular preponderance. Right atrial enlargement is rare. There may be different types of cardiac arrhythmias.

Tricuspid Stenosis

In the absence of atrial fibrillation there is a tall (more than 2·5 mm.) and widened (more than 0·1 sec.) P wave; there is no evidence of right ventricular dominance. Cardiac arrhythmias may be present.

Pulmonary Incompetence

There is usually right ventricular preponderance with or without asymmetrical inversion of the T waves from V_1 to V_3. Right atrium may be enlarged especially when there is congestive cardiac failure.

Pulmonary Stenosis

There may be right ventricular hypertrophy usually with strain (tall R wave in V_1 with inversion of the T wave from V_1 to V_3). In mild cases the electrocardiogram may be normal. There may be tall and peaked P waves.

CHAPTER XI

HYPERTENSIVE HEART DISEASE

The electrocardiogram may be normal in mild cases. In moderate and severe cases there may be a high voltage of the R wave with or without a small Q wave in V_5 and V_6 and equivalent leads; the R wave may be wider than normal (0·11 sec.).

In the early stages there may be simply a high voltage R wave in the left ventricular surface leads; later a high voltage R wave may be associated with a slight depression of the S–T segment with asymmetrical inversion of the T waves in V_5 and V_6 and equivalent leads; this happens when there is left ventricular dilatation with a labouring left ventricle (i.e., with a little or absence of reserve power of the left ventricle).

In V_1 and V_2 leads there is usually a deep S wave with a small R wave, elevated S–T segment and upright T wave (Fig. 95).

A left axis deviation and a horizontal lie are common. When the heart is rotated clockwise the transitional zone is shifted to the right of lead V_4 and when it is rotated

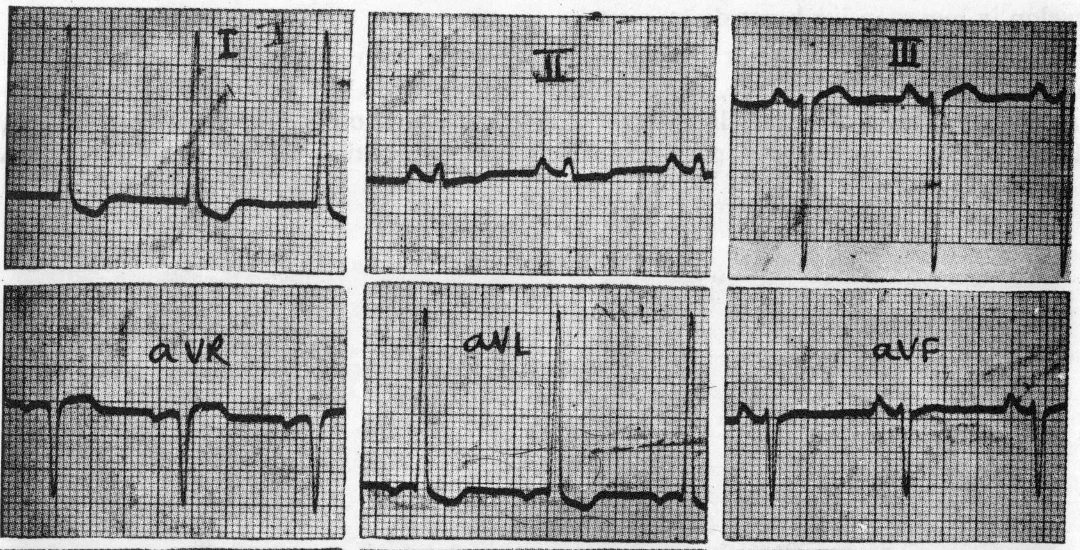

Fig. 95.

Fig. 95 is an electrocardiogram from a case of severe hypertension showing gross left ventricular hypertrophy and strain; the patient was not digitalised.

anticlockwise the transitional zone is shifted to the left of lead V_4 and large R waves with inverted T waves may be seen in lead V_3.

In some cases there may be a vertical lie when the diaphragm is low as in emphysema.

When the heart is vertical lead aVF shows a taller R wave than the depth of the S wave and lead aVL shows a deeper S wave than the height of the R wave. Standard leads in such cases indicate right axis deviation and T wave inversion in leads II and III.

In the standard leads there may be a concordant type of left ventricular hypertrophy, i.e., a tall R wave in all the three standard leads with practically no S wave, and usually with asymmetrical inversion of the T wave.

The larger the size of the left ventricle the higher the amplitude of the R wave in V_5 and V_6, and deeper the amplitude of the S wave in V_1.

There may be a horizontal depression of the S–T segment and inversion of the T wave if there is a complicating ischaemic heart disease.

There may be left bundle-branch block and different degrees of heart block.

Cardiac arrhythmias such as atrial fibrillation, paroxysmal tachycardia, etc., may develop in hypertensive heart disease.

When hypertensive heart disease is complicated with cerebral vascular accidents such as cerebral haemorrhage, subarachnoid haemorrhage, cerebral thrombosis, hypertensive encephalopathy, etc., the electrocardiogram may show a prolonged Q–T interval (duration) and an inversion of a wide T wave in addition to the changes already mentioned.

CHAPTER XII

PULMONARY HYPERTENSION

The term 'Pulmonary Hypertension' is used when there is a high rise of blood pressure in the pulmonary arteries which should be above 30/15 mm. of Hg. The pulmonary hypertension develops when there is obliteration of more than two-thirds of the total cross-section of the pulmonary vascular bed or when there is a gross elevation of the left atrial pressure or when the pulmonary blood flow is about three times or more the normal pulmonary blood flow.

In the electrocardiogram the height of the P wave is more than 2·5 mm. (P pulmonale) and there is a right ventricular preponderance (a tall R wave in V_1, i.e., the height of R wave is 12 mm. or more in case of a large S wave in V_1 or it is at least 7 mm. in height when there is a negligible S wave in V_1) with or without asymmetrical inversion of the T wave from V_1 to V_3 which indicates some degree of right ventricular dilatation with loss of reserve power and impaired function of the right ventricle.

There may be right axis deviation and vertical lie.

In some cases of pulmonary heart disease there may be rS pattern (small R wave with deep S wave) in the chest leads.

An asymmetrical inversion of the T wave may be reversible in the early stage if it occurs during exacerbation of chronic lung disease, such as after an infection or after severe exertion or after severe bronchospasm.

There may be a right bundle-branch block.

In the limb leads the QRS complexes may be of low voltage.

In emphysema the descent of the diaphragm giving rise to a low position of the heart, may give rise to a QS pattern (no R wave) in leads V_3 and V_4, although in the lower intercostal spaces in the V_3 and V_4 lead position and in leads V_5 and V_6 there may be rS patterns.

In emphysema a left axis deviation may be found because of the more vertical direction of the electrical forces or because of associated ischaemic heart disease.

There may be ectopic beats of any type, paroxysmal tachycardia, atrial flutter or fibrillation in some cases. Heart block specially with paroxysmal tachycardia may occasionally be found even without digitalis.

Massive Pulmonary Embolism or Acute Cor pulmonale

Massive pulmonary embolism gives rise to acute pulmonary hypertension. In the electrocardiogram there will be sinus tachycardia; the P wave is increased in height (P pulmonale); there may be transient cardiac arrhythmias such as atrial fibrillation or flutter; occasionally there may be heart block of various degrees.

In standard lead I there should be a deep S wave, and in standard lead III there should be a deep Q wave with an inverted T wave. A marked clockwise rotation may be present; there may be incomplete right bundle-branch block. Acute right ventricular dilatation causes asymmetrical inversion of the T wave and incomplete right bundle-branch block pattern in the right ventricular surface leads.

An S–T segment depression and T wave inversion in the standard lead I and in left ventricular surface leads occur due to coronary insufficiency following a severe and sudden fall in the cardiac output as a result of massive obstruction in the pulmonary circulation; this is more often observed in advanced age.

Occasionally in massive pulmonary embolism the electrocardiogram may resemble postero-inferior myocardial infarction; thus there may occasionally be deep Q waves with inverted T waves in leads II, III and aVF; the deep Q waves in such cases are, however, transient and are predominant in the standard lead III than in aVF; S–T segment elevation is not seen; the T wave inversion in the right ventricular surface leads are not accompanied by deep Q waves or S–T segment elevation in these leads.

CHAPTER XIII

PERICARDITIS AND PERICARDIAL EFFUSION

In pericarditis there is injury to the superficial layers of the myocardium which develop a negative potential. In the initial stage there is elevation of the S–T segment in all the leads; the S–T segment, however, remains concave upwards; there is no abnormal Q wave (Fig. 96).

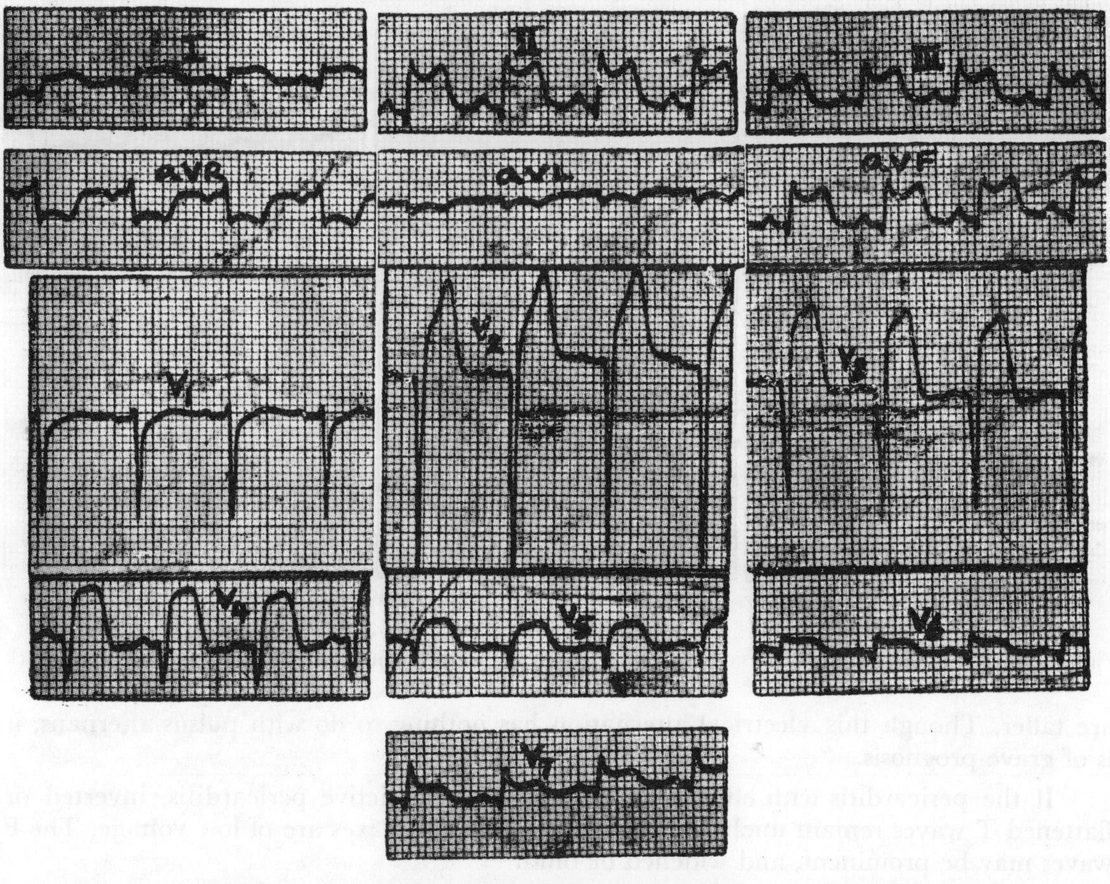

Fig. 96.

Fig. 96 is an electrocardiogram from a case of acute myocardial infarction with localised pericarditis over the postero-inferior wall taken on the 5th day of the clinical attack.

After a few days the S–T segment reaches the base line; it may even be depressed; the T wave is flattened or biphasic or inverted. When the inflammation subsides and there is complete resolution, the T wave becomes upright (Fig. 97).

Pericarditis may be localised when only the corresponding leads show the characteristic changes; thus the changes may be maximum in lead I or III.

If there is pericardial effusion the QRS complexes are of low voltage; besides, the electrocardiogram may show electrical alternation where the alternate QRS complexes

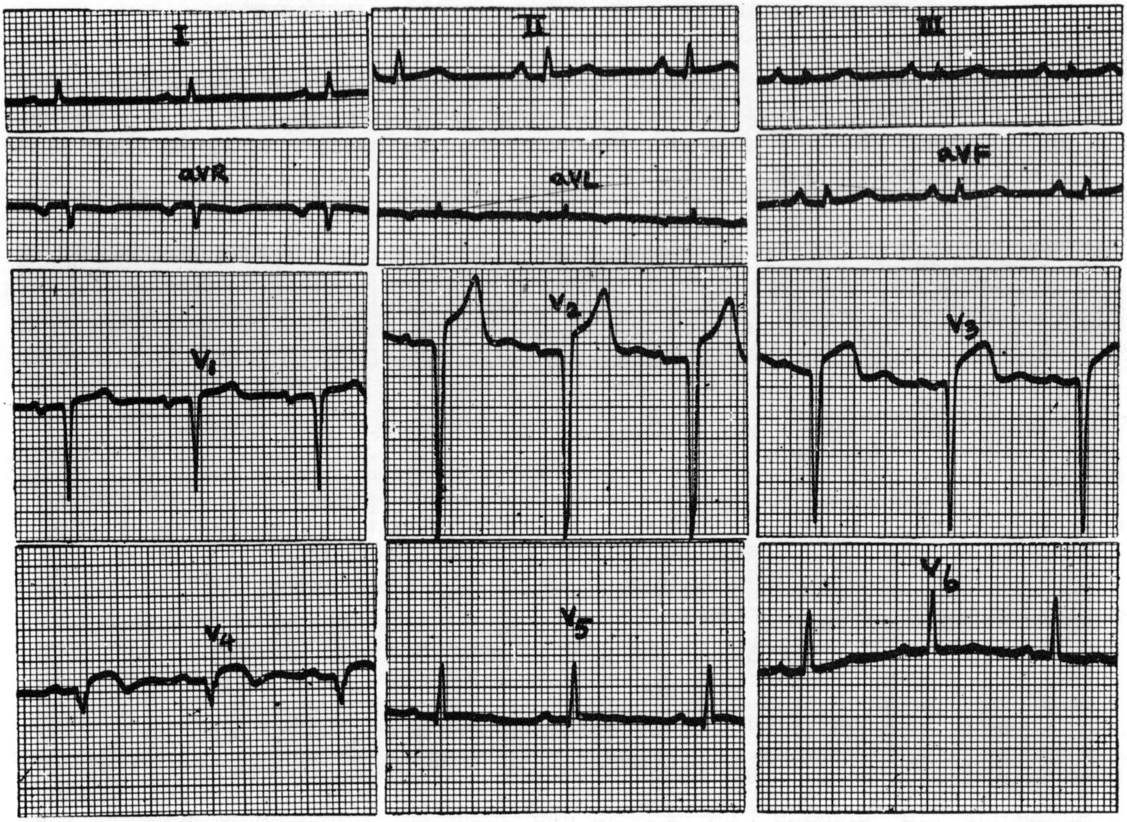

Fig. 97.

Fig. 97 is an electrocardiogram of the same patient as in Fig. 96, taken 8 months after the onset of the clinical attack.

are taller. Though this electrical alternation has nothing to do with pulsus alternans, it is of grave prognosis.

If the pericarditis with effusion is followed by constrictive pericarditis, inverted or flattened T waves remain unchanged and the QRS complexes are of low voltage. The P waves may be prominent, and widened or bifid.

The diagnosis of pericarditis depends on the characteristic initial changes in the electrocardiogram, changing picture of the QRS–T complexes in the serial electrocardiograms and the characteristic clinical features associated with it.

CHAPTER XIV

ELECTROCARDIOGRAM IN CONGENITAL HEART DISEASE

Foetal Electrocardiography

Maternal and foetal electrocardiograms may be taken with an electrocardiograph fitted with a preamplifier (amplifying 50 times and recording a frequency of 12--20 cycles per second) by means of bipolar leads, one electrode being placed at the level of fundus of the uterus and the other being placed just above the symphysis pubis.

Foetal electrocardiography helps in detecting foetal life, foetal cardiac arrhythmia, and foetal heart rate. It also helps in determining position of the foetus and in detecting multiple pregnancies.

Electrocardiogram in Infancy and Childhood

The heart rate is faster in infancy and childhood. At birth the average heart rate is 120–130/minute; then the rate gradually becomes less and it is about 80/minute at puberty. The P–R interval and the QRS duration are relatively short. There is right axis deviation; tall R waves in the right ventricular surface leads (V_1 and V_2) and deep S waves in the left ventricular surface leads (V_5 and V_6) are common findings until the 2nd year of life; occasionally there may be a right bundle-branch block pattern in the electrocardiogram in a normal child. In infancy the inversion of the T wave may be found in the first four chest leads, i.e., from V_1 to V_4. In the unipolar limb leads and in the standard leads large T waves may be found.

It is interesting to note that the T wave is upward in V_1 and V_2, and downward in V_5 and V_6 for the first 24 hours after birth; on about the 4th day of life the T wave becomes inverted in V_1 and V_2, and upright in V_5 and V_6.

The lie of the heart is vertical in infants.

The P wave in aVL may be deeper than that in aVR.

In aVR there may be an occasional upright T wave, and a tall R wave.

In aVF a small Q wave and a large R wave is usually found; in aVF there is frequently a flat or inverted T wave.

Electrocardiogram in Congenital Heart Disease

In congenital heart disease the electrocardiogram is very helpful as it provides a corroborative evidence for diagnosis.

The congenital heart disease may be grouped under two broad headings:

1. Those with a shunt.
2. Those without a shunt.

Congenital Heart Disease with a Shunt

Cyanotic form of Ebstein's disease

In this malformation there is an anomaly of the tricuspid valve and the upper part of right ventricular wall. The posterior leaflet is mostly malformed and is attached to the ventricular endocardium over an wide area.

There is an enlargement of the right atrium which is very characteristic in intracardiac electrocardiogram from the right atrium. There is also right bundle-branch block.

There may be conduction disturbances such as wide and notched P wave with an increased P–R interval, intraventricular conduction defect, etc. In V_1 and in V_2 or even in V_3 there may be low voltage QRS complexes. The shape of QRS complexes may alter from time to time due to a change in the pathway of excitation wave due to the anomalous structure of right ventricle.

In some cases the electrocardiogram may be normal.

Atrial septal defect

An incomplete or complete right bundle-branch block is seen in about 95% of the cases; this is due to a dilatation and prolonged activation of the right ventricle (Fig. 98).

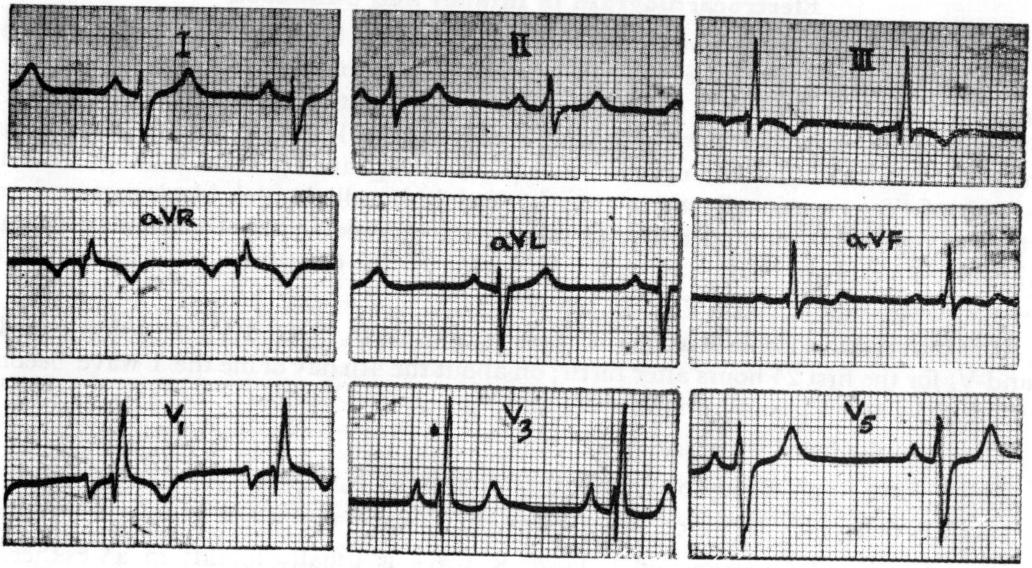

Fig. 98.

Fig. 98 in an electrocardiogram from a female patient aged 21 years who had atrial septal defect; the tracing shows incomplete right bundle-branch block and right ventricular strain.

The P wave is normal in uncomplicated cases. The increased height of the P wave may be due to the presence of an associated pulmonary stenosis or an increased pulmonary vascular resistance.

The P–R interval may be prolonged.

Atrial fibrillation may be present but its incidence is greater with advancing age of the patient.

In ostium primum defects the electrocardiogram shows a left axis deviation, widened P wave, prolonged P–R interval along with right bundle-branch block. The electrical axis may be altered if there is an associated pulmonary stenosis or increased pulmonary vascular resistance. In the standard lead II a split or notched S wave is suggestive of ostium primum defect. There may be an evidence of left ventricular hypertrophy or biventricular hypertrophy in the precordial leads in ostium primum defect.

Ventricular septal defect

The electrocardiogram may be normal in case of small defects (Maladie de Roger).

In case of moderate and large defects the electrocardiogram may show QR pattern in the leads V_5 and V_6, Q wave being a significant one; there may be inversion of the T wave and the U wave (when present) in V_5 and V_6. Heart block is rare (Fig. 99).

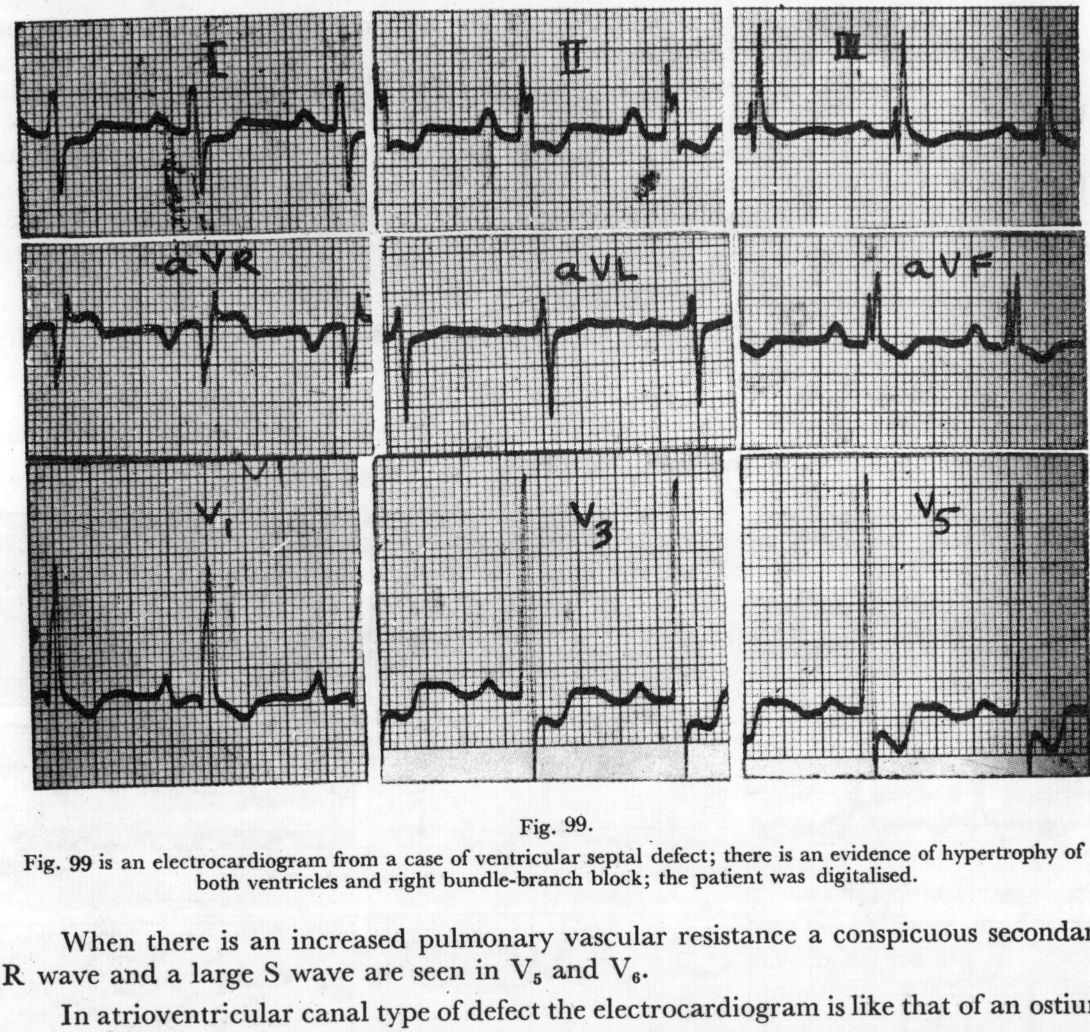

Fig. 99.

Fig. 99 is an electrocardiogram from a case of ventricular septal defect; there is an evidence of hypertrophy of both ventricles and right bundle-branch block; the patient was digitalised.

When there is an increased pulmonary vascular resistance a conspicuous secondary R wave and a large S wave are seen in V_5 and V_6.

In atrioventricular canal type of defect the electrocardiogram is like that of an ostium primum defect.

In rare instances of ventricular septal defect between the left ventricle and the right atrium the electrocardiogram may show evidences of enlargement of right atrium and both ventricles with or without conduction defects.

Patent ductus arteriosus

The electrocardiogram tracing may be normal in many cases; in case of large shunts a significant Q wave with a large R wave may be found in V_5 and V_6 leads often with an inverted U wave: the T wave may be inverted in some cases of large shunts in the left ventricular surface leads. In infants there may be an evidence of right ventricular hypertrophy as well.

Eisenmenger's syndrome

In the electrocardiogram the P wave may be normal in about half of the cases; the P wave is increased in height in others; rarely the P wave may be widened as well especially in patent ductus arteriosus.

A large Q wave is usually seen in V_5 and V_6 leads in patent ductus arteriosus and less commonly in ventricular septal defects.

A large R wave in V_1 is commonly seen when there is atrial septal defect but may be absent in others.

In majority of the cases with patent ductus arteriosus there may be an evidence of enlargement of both the ventricles.

A large R wave and a large S wave are usually found in the chest leads in ventricular septal defect.

Fallot's tetralogy

The P wave is increased in height in about one-third of the cases; thus in majority of the cases the P wave is normal.

A right axis deviation is a common feature.

The QRS deflection in lead V_1 shows a slight to severe degree of right ventricular dominance in about 97% of the cases (Fig.100).

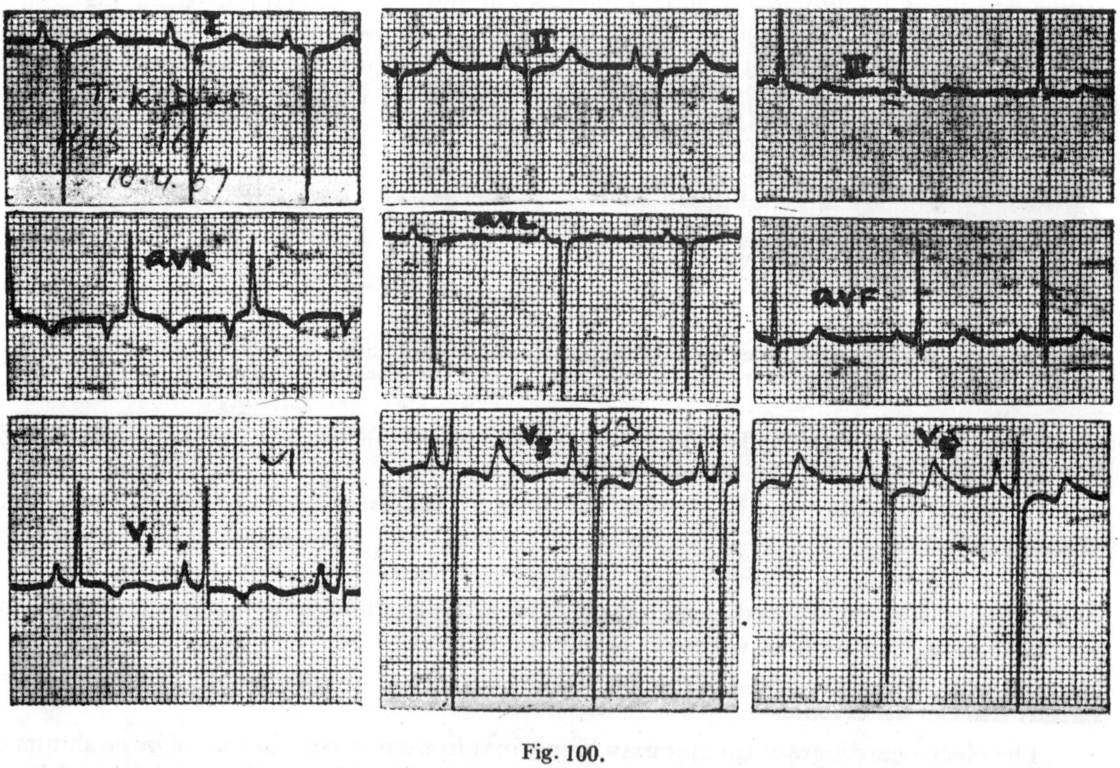

Fig. 100.

Fig.100 is an electrocardiogram of a male patient aged 12 years who had Fallot's tetralogy. Here is an evidence of enlargement of right atrium and right ventricle, right axis, vertical lie, and marked clockwise rotation; there is also some degree of right ventricular strain.

Exceptionally there may be an increased intrinsicoid deflection and inversion of T wave in V_1.

Pulmonary atresia

The electrocardiographic features are similar to those found in Fallot's tetralogy.

Tricuspid atresia

In this there is also a defective development of right ventricle as well.

In the electrocardiogram a large P pulmonale is a dominant feature and an evidence of the left ventricular hypertrophy is usually seen. There is usually a left axis deviation except in young infants.

Aortic septal defect

In this type there is a failure of full development of the spiral septum inside the truncus arteriosus in its basal portion giving rise to a congenital aortopulmonary fistula.

In the electrocardiogram there is an evidence of enlargement of both ventricles. Thus there may be a tall R wave and a deep S wave in all the precordial leads.

Lutembacher's syndrome

In this type of malformation there is a gross atrial septal defect along with mitral stenosis; this is accompanied by a marked dilatation of the pulmonary artery with a left-sided chest deformity.

In the electrocardiogram there may be a prolonged P–R interval, an widened QRS complex and an RSR′ pattern of QRS complex in V_1; the electrocardiogram may show evidence of right ventricular hypertrophy and strain; left atrial enlargement is not usually seen.

Common atrioventricular canal

Here there is incomplete development of the atrial and ventricular septa together with formation of a single atrioventricular valve as a result of fusion of the maldeveloped mitral and tricuspid valves due to arrest in the development of the heart. If there is also gross septal defect at both atrial and ventricular levels there is virtually a single atrium and a single ventricle communicating through a common canal guarded by a single atrioventricular valve.

In the electrocardiogram there is usually a right axis deviation and an evidence of hypertrophy of both ventricles. There may be a complete or partial heart block.

Aneurysm of sinus of Valsalva rupturing into the right atrium or right ventricle or pulmonary artery

This results from a congenital weakness of the base of the aorta due to hypoplasia. The aneurysm develops after birth and eventually ruptures into right ventricle, right atrium or pulmonary artery. The aneurysm of sinus of Valsalva may, however, be of syphilitic or mycotic origin, in addition to congenital cause.

In the electrocardiogram there may be an intraventricular conduction defect and an evidence of left ventricular or biventricular hypertrophy, depending on the site of rupture of the sinus of Valsalva.

Pulmonary stenosis with atrial or ventricular septal defect

When Pulmonary stenosis is associated with a reversed shunt the electrocardiogram shows an evidence of gross right ventricular and right atrial enlargement.

When pulmonary stenosis is associated with a left to right shunt the electrocardiogram does not usually show any evidence of right atrial and right ventricular enlargement.

Transposition of the great vessels

In the electrocardiogram there is evidence of gross hypertrophy of the right ventricle usually a few weeks after birth. There is usually a right axis deviation.

If there is an associated ventricular septal defect there may be evidence of hypertrophy of both the ventricles.

If there is an associated tricuspid atresia or single ventricle there may be an evidence of left ventricular hypertrophy and left axis deviation.

Persistent truncus arteriosus

In this malformation there is failure of development of the aortic septum inside the primitive aortic sac; the common truncus overrides the ventricular septum; there is a high ventricular septal defect. The orifice of the truncus possesses 2 or 3 or 4 or more semilunar valve cusps and the pulmonary artery arises from the truncus.

Presence of hypertrophy of both ventricles, and that of right atrium are the usual findings. In some cases there may be right ventricular hypertrophy or right atrial hypertrophy alone. There may be normal or right axis of the atria.

In hemitruncus arteriosus one pulmonary artery originates from the truncus and the other pulmonary artery arises directly from the right ventricle. The electrocardiogram is usually normal in this case.

Total anomalous pulmonary venous drainage

The electrocardiographic features depend on the associated lesions such as patent foramen ovale, ostium secundum atrial septal defect, patent ductus arteriosus, single atrium, etc.

There is usually a right axis deviation, right atrial and right ventricular hypertrophy, and incomplete right bundle-branch block; a QR pattern with a deep S wave in the left ventricular surface leads may indicate presence of the associated lesions as mentioned.

Anomalous drainage of superior or inferior vena cava into left atrium

In the electrocardiogram there may be a deep S wave in V_2 which may be 25 mm. or more; there may be an evidence of left ventricular hypertrophy.

Double outlet right ventricle

In this both aorta and pulmonary artery arise from the right ventricle; pulmonary orifice is usually constricted with or without a bicuspid valve; there is also a ventricular septal defect.

In the electrocardiogram a right axis deviation, an evidence of right ventricular hypertrophy and strain and a high and peaked P wave are found.

Defective development of right ventricle with absence of ventricular septal defect

In this the right ventricle remains as a small chamber with a stenosed pulmonary valve orifice and a diminutive pulmonary artery; a small tricuspid orifice opens into the small right ventricle.

In the electrocardiogram a right axis deviation may be present; an evidence of right ventricular hypertrophy is very uncommon; an evidence of left ventricular hypertrophy may be found; a very tall and peaked P wave is very suggestive of this malformation (Fig.101).

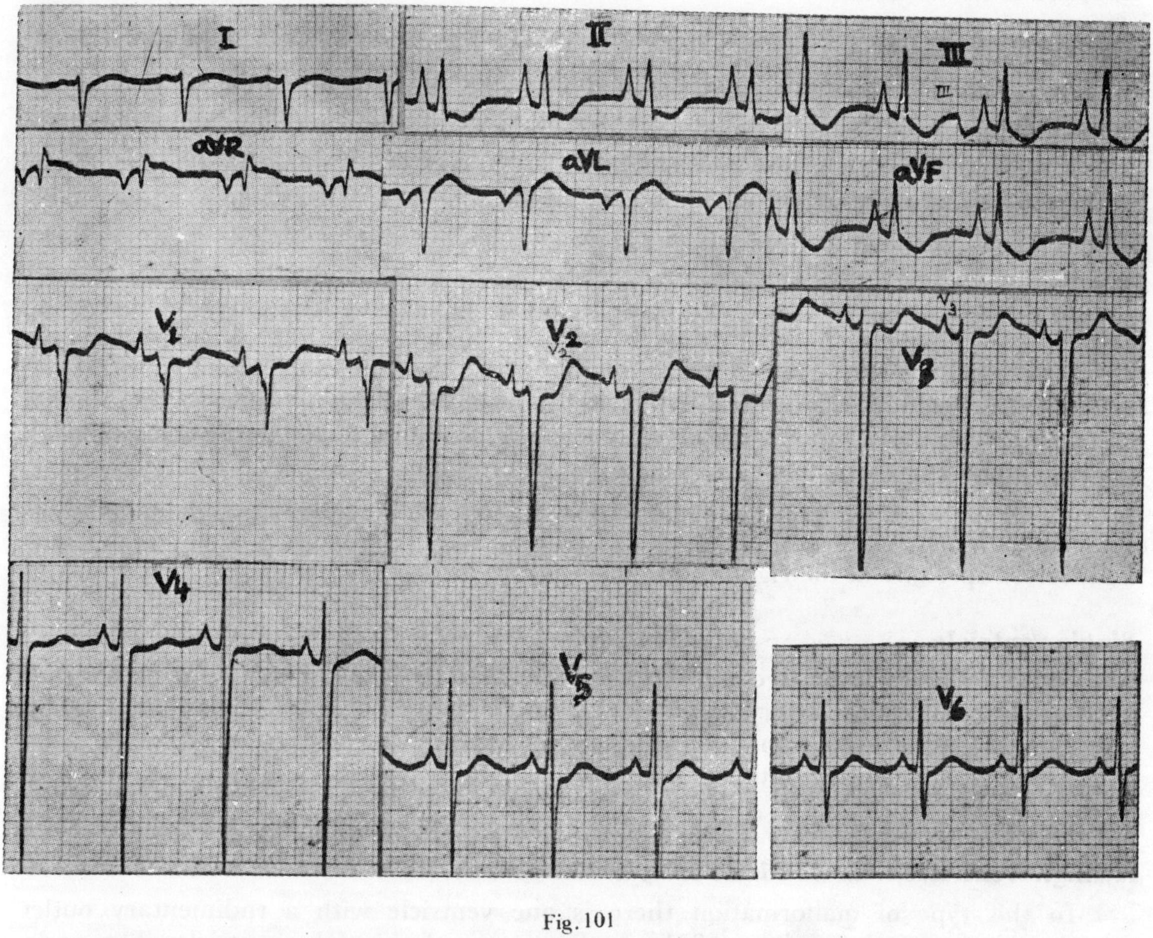

Fig. 101

Fig. 101 shows a huge right atrium and absence of right ventricular hypertrophy in a case of congenital small right ventricle.

Parchment right ventricle

In this there is defective development of the musculature of the right ventricle. The right ventricle is relatively large and thin-walled containing little heart muscle.

In the electrocardiogram P wave may be abnormally high and evidence of left ventricular dominance may be present.

Taussig-Bing malformation

In this type of malformation the aorta arises from the right ventricle and lies to the right of the pulmonary artery which also arises mainly from the right ventricle. The pulmonary artery, however, overrides the ventricular septum and receives blood also from the left ventricle. A high ventricular septal defect is present. The aorta is smaller or normal in size but the pulmonary artery is usually large.

In the electrocardiogram a right axis deviation and an evidence of right ventricular hypertrophy are seen.

Absence of aortic arch

In this type of congenital malformation there is complete interruption of isthmus region of the aorta. The ductus arteriosus remains patent and communicates with the descending aorta. The cyanosis is present in the lower limbs and extends up to the brim of the pelvis.

A right axis deviation and an evidence of right ventricular hypertrophy are present in the electrocardiogram.

Aortic atresia with hypoplasia of ascending aorta

In this malformation there is atresia of aortic valve with hypoplasia of ascending aorta and aortic arch up to the site of entrance of ductus arteriosus. There is also defective development of the left ventricle which interferes with the outflow of blood from the left atrium. An associated atrial septal defect is common. The systemic flow is maintained chiefly by blood flow from left atrium to the right atrium and finally to the aorta through the right ventricle, pulmonary artery and ductus arteriosus.

In the electrocardiogram a right axis deviation and an evidence of gross right ventricular hypertrophy and strain are obtained. The T wave may be small and may be inverted specially in the right ventricular surface leads.

Single ventricle

This is usually associated with transposition of the great vessels, and stenosis or atresia of the pulmonary artery.

The electrocardiogram may show features of hypertrophy of single or both ventricles, a normal or right axis deviation; there may be a deep Q wave and a tall R wave in leads V_1 and V_2.

A single ventricle with a rudimentary outlet chamber

In this type of malformation there is one ventricle with a rudimentary outlet chamber occupying the position of the outflow tract of the right ventricle. The aorta usually arises from the common ventricle and the pulmonary artery from the rudimentary chamber.

In the electrocardiogram there may be a right axis or a left axis deviation. There is a deep S wave from V_1 to V_6 in case of left axis deviation. Again there may be an evidence of left ventricular hypertrophy in V leads with a right axis deviation (Fig.102).

Congenital Heart Disease without a Shunt

Familial cardiomyopathy

In the Evans type where there is enlargement of the left ventricle specially, the electrocardiogram shows a large R wave with inverted T wave in the left ventricular surface leads and their equivalents; there may be left bundle-branch block; atrial fibrillation or paroxysmal tachycardia or complete heart block are occasional findings.

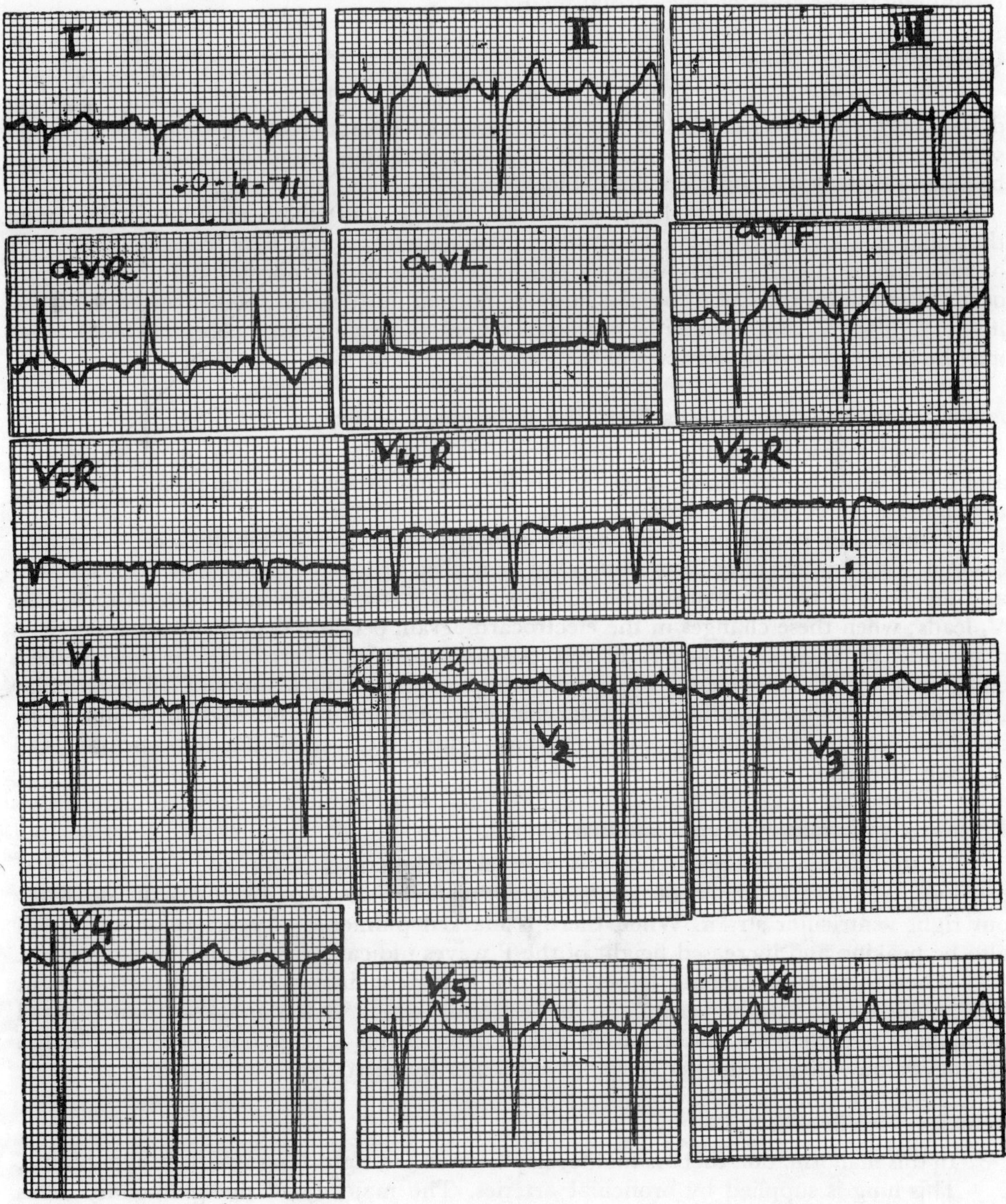

Fig.102.

Fig.102 is an electrocardiogram from a proved case of single ventricle with transposition of great vessels and pulmonary stenosis; the patient was a lady aged 18 years who had gross cyanosis and clubbing.

In familial cardiomyopathy with asymmetrical hypertrophy of the heart and inflow tract obstruction the electrocardiogram shows a conspicuous Q wave and inversion of the T wave with or without elevation of the S–T segment in leads II, III and aVF resembling posteroinferior myocardial infarction.

Congenital heart block

This may be associated with Evans type of familial cardiomyopathy, ostium primum defect, corrected transposition of the great vessels or exceptionally with the ventricular septal defect. There may be increased P–R interval, left bundle-branch block, right bundle-branch block, complete heart block, etc.

In congenital complete heart block the resting ventricular rate is usually faster than that in acquired complete heart block; the ventricular rate may increase after effort or injection of atropine; very rarely a normal rhythm with a normal P–R interval may occur after effort; the QRS complex may be normal in duration; and inverted T waves, if any, in leads V_5 and V_6 may be corrected on exertion; congenital complete heart block may be present in other members of the family.

A left coronary artery arising from the pulmonary artery

In such a case the right coronary artery which arises as usual from the aorta, is large and feeds both the ventricles, a retrograde flow being present into the pulmonary artery through the left coronary artery.

If there are symptoms of ischaemia and dyspnoea which usually occur between 6 weeks and 12 weeks after birth there may be a deep Q wave, elevation of S–T segment and inversion of the T wave suggesting myocardial infarction specially in I, aVL, V_5 and V_6 leads; when these changes in the electrocardiogram occur and persist in infancy it is diagnostic of anomalous origin of left coronary artery. There may be low voltage complexes and T wave changes in standard leads; there are no features of left ventricular hypertrophy as it is only dilated. Those who escape the features of myocardial infarction in infancy and reach adult life may only show evidence of ventricular hypertrophy, and T wave inversion.

Primary pulmonary hypertension

In the electrocardiogram there is a marked right axis deviation. The precordial leads may show an evidence of marked right ventricular hypertrophy with or without right ventricular strain. When there is marked pulmonary hypertension there will also be peaking and increased height of the P waves indicating right atrial enlargement.

When there is pulmonary hypertension with patent ductus arteriosus there is right axis deviation with right ventricular hypertrophy which is less marked than isolated pulmonary hypertension. If the patent ductus arteriosus is a large one there may be left axis deviation with an evidence of right ventricular hypertrophy.

Scimitar syndrome

In this malformation there is maldevelopment of the right lung which is hypoplastic.

This lung is supplied by bronchial arteries. The majority of the pulmonary veins of this lung unite to form a common vessel which enters the inferior vena cava after passing through the diaphragm.

The electrocardiogram is normal.

Glycogen storage disease

In this disease there is a large deposition of glycogen in cardiac and striated muscles as a result of congenital defect of carbohydrate metabolism. This may run in a family. The wall of the ventricles may be enormously thickened and the heart is considerably enlarged.

In the electrocardiogram P–R interval may be shortened with a slight prolongation of the QRS complex which is large with a depression of S–T segment and an inversion of the T wave; a very high voltage R wave and a deep inverted T wave with a prominent Q wave in leads I, V_5 and V_6 may be seen; rarely W. P. W. syndrome may be found. These changes are not usually present at birth but they develop after a few months.

Congenital mitral stenosis

This may occur as an isolated anomaly or in combination with other congenital anomalies. Mitral stenosis or mitral incompetence or both may be present.

In the electrocardiogram there is a right axis deviation and an evidence of right ventricular dominance. The P wave may be wide and notched and the P–R interval may be prolonged.

Coronary arteriovenous fistulae

The electrocardiogram may suggest acute myocardial infarction of postero-inferior wall without any evidence of healing. There may be an evidence of left ventricular hypertrophy.

Endocardial fibro-elastosis

This is found in infants and is said to be congenital in origin due to a developmental anomaly of the endocardium which is rendered white, smooth and thickened. There is an excessive growth of collagen and elastic tissue beneath the endocardial lining. This may involve one or more than one or all chambers of the heart often with abnormalities of the mitral and aortic valves.

The electrocardiogram may show an evidence of left ventricular hypertrophy, viz., a tall R wave with an inverted T wave in V_5 and V_6.

Congenital aneurysmal dilatation of left atrium

This is very rare. The electrocardiogram may show small P waves which may be inverted in standard lead I and upright in standard leads II and III.

Corrected transposition of great vessels

In this type the aorta is situated to the left and anterior to the pulmonary artery. The aorta receives arterial blood coming from the left atrium and the pulmonary artery receives venous blood coming from the right atrium. There is a transposition of the ventricles and that of the mitral and tricuspid valves so that the mitral valve directs the blood flow from the right atrium into the pulmonary ventricle which possesses the anatomical features of the left ventricle and the tricuspid valve directs the blood flow from the left atrium into the systemic ventricle which possesses anatomical features of the right ventricle and gives origin to the aorta. Coronary arteries are also abnormal.

The electrocardiogram may show a tall P wave and partial or complete heart block; a QR pattern may be seen in leads III, aVR and aVF indicating left ventricular hypertrophy; a QR pattern may also be seen in V_1 along with an RS pattern in V_5 and V_6. A marked accentuation of the second heart sound over the pulmonary area along with evidences of biventricular hypertrophy, left being greater than right, is suspicious of corrected transposition of the great vessels.

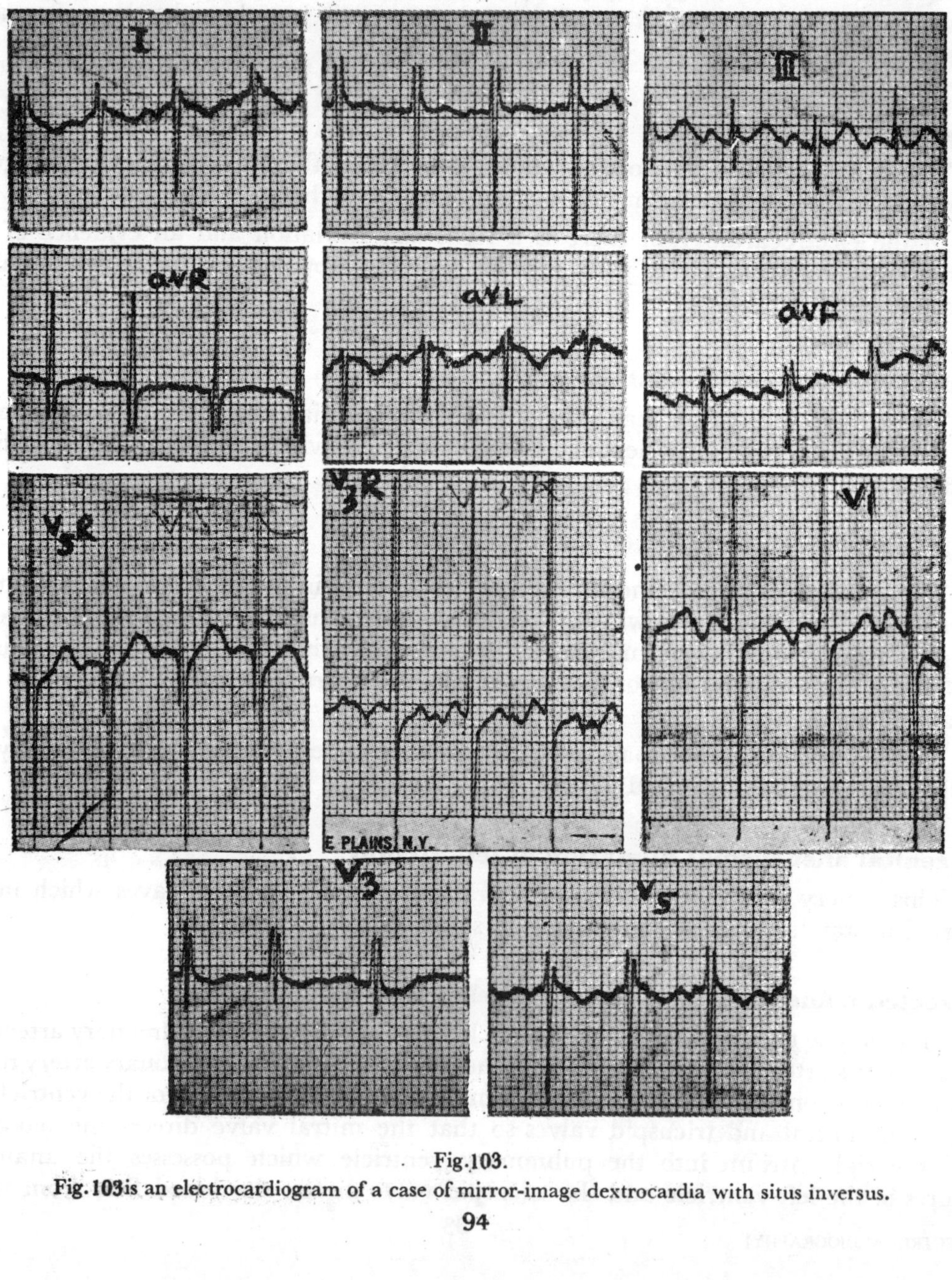

Fig.103.

Fig. 103 is an electrocardiogram of a case of mirror-image dextrocardia with situs inversus.

Dextrocardia with situs inversus

In this condition the primitive cardiac loop swings in a reverse direction and the position of all the organs of the body is the mirror image of the normal situation.

In the electrocardiogram the standard lead I shows inversion of both P and T waves with the QRS deflection being mirror image of the normal; the standard leads II and III replace each other; leads aVR and aVL also replace each other. In case of unipolar precordial leads V_1, V_2, V_3, V_4, V_5 and V_6 in a normally placed heart will be equivalent to or represented by V_2L (i.e., 4th left intercostal space near the sternal margin), V_1R (i.e., 4th right intercostal space near the sternal margin), V_3R, V_4R, V_5R and V_6R respectively in a case of dextrocardia, that is, the leads have to be placed on the right side of the chest to get the equivalent tracing.

Thus in precordial leads on the left side there is lack of gradual increase in the height of the R wave as we get normally from V_1 to V_6; on the right side, i.e., from V_1 to V_6R the height of the R wave gradually increases which is not seen in a normal electrocardiogram (Fig.103).

Dextrorotation of the heart or Dextroversion

In this abnormality the primitive cardiac loop swings incompletely to the right. This is usually associated with gross malformations of the heart along with frequent abnormalities of other thoracic and abdominal viscerae.

In dextrorotation of the heart there is an inversion of the P waves in standard leads II and III probably indicating an abnormal origin of the pacemaker of the heart; the P waves in standard lead I is, however, upright and the T wave is inverted. The unipolar chest leads V_2L and V_3L or simply V_2 and V_3 represent deflections of the anterior chamber, and V_5R and V_6R represent deflections of the posterior chamber.

Situs inversus with laevocardia (Fig.104)

In situs inversus of this type there is a transposition of the atria as well as that of the great vessels with the heart rotating back to a position on the left side of the chest; thus the right atrium opens into the left ventricle from which the pulmonary artery arises; the left atrium directs the blood into the right ventricle from which the aorta arises; the inferior vena cava lies on the left under such circumstances with the persistence of the left superior vena cava. The inferior vena cava may, however, be absent and the venous drainage of the lower limbs may then take place through the azygos system of veins.

The electrocardiogram may sometimes be normal. There may be an inversion of the P waves in standard leads. Different types of cardiac arrhythmias are usually present.

Coarctation of the aorta

The electrocardiogram may be normal in almost half of the cases. In others there may be evidence of left ventricular hypertrophy with or without strain; gross hypertrophy of the left ventricle may occur when this is associated with aortic stenosis or regurgitation, mitral regurgitation, patent ductus arteriosus, ventricular septal defect, etc. Rarely there may be right bundle-branch block.

In early infancy there is usually a right axis deviation and an evidence of right ventricular hypertrophy.

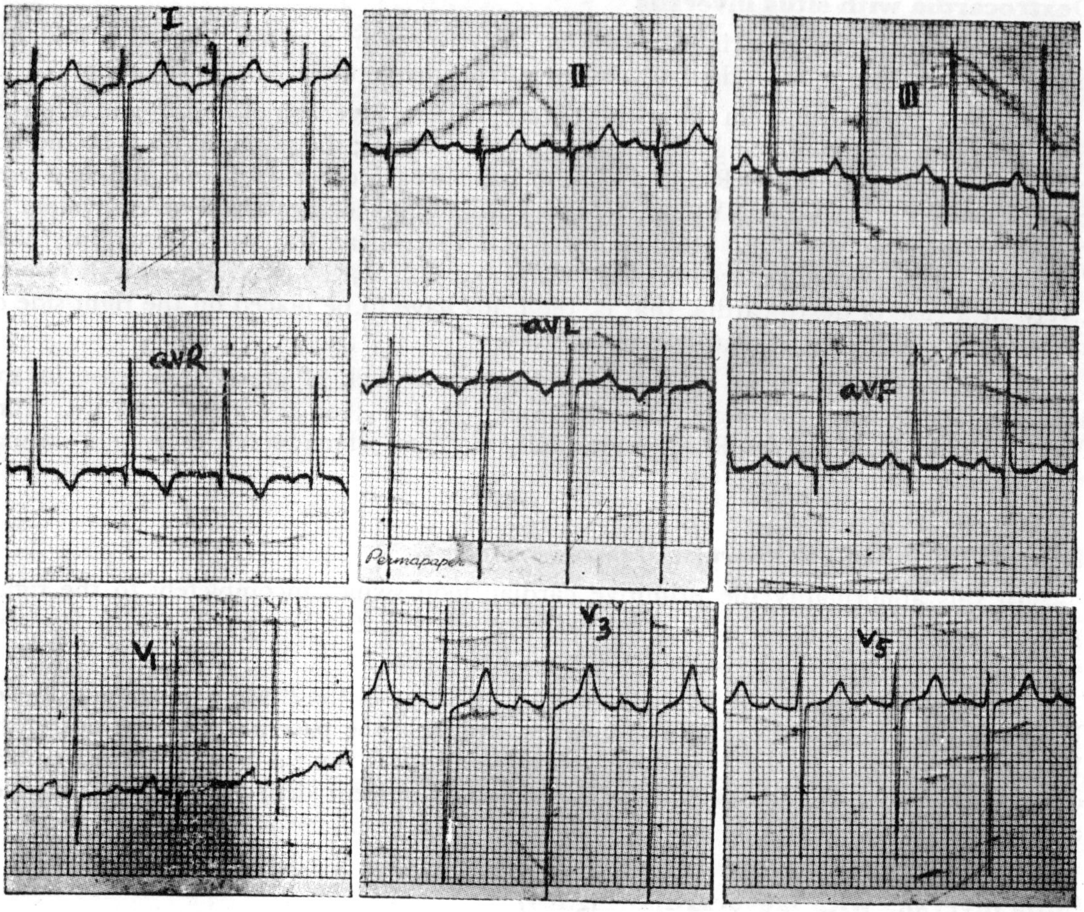

Fig.104.

Fig.104 is an electrocardiogram from a proved case of laevocardia with transposition of great vessels.

Aortic valve stenosis

There may be evidence of left ventricular hypertrophy (tall R wave in V_5 and V_6 or equivalent leads) with or without strain (asymmetrical inversion of the T wave) with or without S–T segment depression. There may be a prolonged intrinsicoid deflection in left ventricular surface leads.

In mild and moderate stenosis the electrocardiogram is frequently normal.

There is a right axis deviation in infancy and early childhood.

Supra-aortic stenosis

The appearance is similar to that in aortic stenosis (*vide* supra).

High subvalvular membrane stenosis

In the electrocardiogram there is usually a high voltage R wave with deep asymmetrical inversion of the T wave with or without depression of the S–T segment in V_5 and V_6 and their equivalent leads.

Subvalvular fibrous ring stenosis

The electrocardiogram tracing is similar in appearance to that found in high subvalvular membrane stenosis.

Left ventricular obstructive cardiomyopathy

In this type of cardiomyopathy there may be a tall R wave with or without a small Q wave, flattened, biphasic or asymmetrical inversion of the T wave in V_5, V_6 and their equivalent leads; S–T segment depression may be found in some cases; there may be occasionally left bundle-branch block, and cardiac arrhythmias.

Congenital mitral regurgitation

Congenital mitral regurgitation which may occur as a result of absence of the chordae tendineae, cleft mitral valve, or overburdened left ventricle, may show a tall R wave with a small Q wave, asymmetrical inversion of the T wave, with or without depression of the S–T segment in V_5, V_6 or their equivalent leads.

Cor triatriatum

In this case there are three chambers in the atrial side, the left atrium being divided by an anomalous transverse septum which develops a small aperture establishing communication between the two pockets of the left atrium, the proximal one receiving the pulmonary veins and the distal one communicating with the left ventricle through a normal mitral orifice.

In the electrocardiogram there is no enlargement of the left atrium; the P wave is, however, peaked with an increased height which indicates right atrial enlargement due to associated increased pulmonary vascular resistance. Right ventricular dominance may be present due to the same reason. A right axis deviation is present.

Idiopathic dilatation of the pulmonary artery

The electrocardiogram is normal; functional pulmonary incompetence may be present and in that case there will be evidence of right ventricular enlargement (tall R wave in V_1) and delayed right ventricular activation (rSR′ pattern of the QRS complex, and the intrinsicoid deflection more than 0·02 sec. in V_1). When there is a gross dilatation of right ventricle, tricuspid incompetence may occur and there will be enlargement of the right atrium (tall and peaked P wave) as well.

Ebstein's anomaly (acyanotic)

In about 90% of the cases there is right bundle-branch block (rSR′ in V_1); the P waves are tall and sharp; the P–R interval may be prolonged; in some cases there may be W.P.W syndrome; the voltage of the QRS complexes may be low.

Isolated pulmonary valvular stenosis

The electrocardiogram shows right ventricular hypertrophy (tall R wave in V_1); there may also be a right ventricular strain pattern; tall P waves indicating right atrial enlargement may also be present; rarely there may be right bundle-branch block.

When the pulmonary stenosis is mild there may only be a right axis deviation.

When it is extreme apart from the changes already mentioned there may be a T wave inversion up to V_5 and a deep S wave in left ventricular surface leads (*vide* Review Tracing 33).

Infundibular stenosis

The electrocardiogram does not usually show any evidence of right ventricular preponderance. There may however be a progressive right ventricular strain which is out of proportion to the size of the heart. The P waves may be both tall and wide.

Pulmonary artery branch stenosis

In the electrocardiogram there may be a right axis deviation and an evidence of right ventricular hypertrophy.

Arteriovenous aneurysm

In this type of vascular anomaly there is usually hypertrophy of both ventricles as a result of hyperkinetic circulation. In the electrocardiogram an increased height of P waves and changes in QRS–T complexes may be seen.

CHAPTER XV

ELECTROCARDIOGRAPHIC CHANGES IN MISCELLANEOUS CONDITIONS

Electrocardiogram as such does not give the diagnosis of a disease. It can, however, confirm or reject a clinical diagnosis, or may suggest a diagnosis when considered with other data.

In this chapter the value of electrocardiogram in the diagnosis of some diseases, and alteration in the electrocardiographic tracing in various diseased conditions have been discussed.

Myxoedema

In uncomplicated myxoedema there is sinus bradycardia with low voltage P–QRS–T complexes; the T wave is low, flat, biphasic or inverted due to associated myocardial changes. Rarely there may be myocardial ischaemia; more rarely myocardial infarction without coronary thrombosis has been reported especially after vigorous treatment with thyroxine. Atrial fibrillation may be present especially when myxoedema develops after thyrotoxicosis.

Thyrotoxicosis

In thyrotoxicosis there is sinus tachycardia. There may be atrial flutter or fibrillation. A high voltage of the P–QRS–T complexes may be seen. An elevation of S–T segment with inversion of T wave may be found usually in left ventricular surface leads (Fig.105).

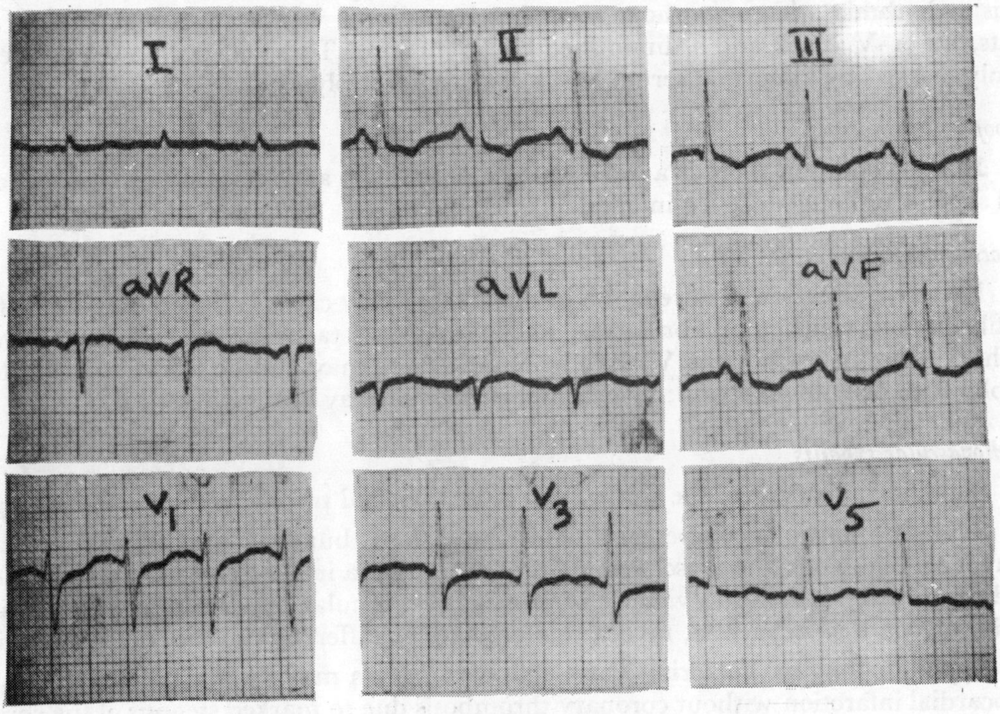

Fig. 105.

Fig.105 is an electrocardiogram from a case of thyrotoxicosis.

Cushing's Syndrome

The electrocardiogram is usually normal. If there is hypertension, the evidence of left ventricular hypertrophy with or without strain may be present. The high serum potassium level may cause a tall and peaked T wave; there may also be widening of the P wave and the QRS complex.

Hyperaldosteronism

The condition is associated with a low level of serum potassium and the features of the same may be seen in the electrocardiogram; thus there may be depression of the S–T segment with low, flat or inverted T wave, prolongation of the P–R and the Q–T intervals, and prominence of the U wave.

Acromegaly

There may be evidence of enlargement of both the ventricles; the T wave may be flat, biphasic or inverted; in some cases myocardial ischaemia may be present due to associated coronary disease.

Addison's disease

The electrocardiogram usually shows evidence of hyperpotassaemia; thus there will be a tall and peaked T wave. Characteristically there may be low voltage complexes.

Hyperparathyroidism

The electrocardiogram may show evidence of hypercalcaemia; thus there may be sinus arrhythmia with or without sinus bradycardia, a wandering pacemaker, ectopic beats, an A–V block and a diminished Q–Tc interval. These effects, however, are commonly masked by abnormal serum levels of other electrolytes.

Hypoparathyroidism

In this condition there is a low serum calcium level and thus the electrocardiogram will show a prolonged Q–Tc interval.

Pheochromocytoma

Excessive secretion of adrenaline in this disease may cause ectopic beats, atrial flutter or fibrillation, ventricular fibrillation, and paroxysmal tachycardias; transient inversion of the T wave in leads V_4 to V_6 may be found; there may also be left ventricular hypertrophy with or without strain; myocardial ischaemia may also be observed.

Cardiovascular syphilis

Syphilitic aneurysm of the aorta: This gives a normal picture in the electrocardiogram.

Syphilitic aortic incompetence: This may show bundle-branch block or various degrees of A–V block due to ischaemic fibrosis or gumma in the myocardium. The electrocardiogram may also show evidence of gross left ventricular hypertrophy with or without strain, myocardial ischaemia, myocardial changes or different varieties of arrhythmias.

Syphilitic Angina Pectoris: The electrocardiogram may show a pattern of a typical myocardial infarction without coronary thrombosis due to marked stenosis of the coronary ostia. There may be evidence of coronary insufficiency, different types of arrhythmias, or ischaemic myocardial changes due to narrowing of the coronary ostia.

Syphilitic heart block: Different types of heart block may occur if the A–V node and the bundle of His are involved directly by a gumma or indirectly by ischaemic fibrosis following coronary insufficiency due to stenosis of the coronary ostia.

Friedreich's Ataxia

The electrocardiogram may show T wave changes; there may also be bundle-branch block or various types of cardiac arrhythmias such as atrial flutter, atrial fibrillation, paroxysmal tachycardias, etc.

Pseudohypertrophic Muscular Dystrophy

The electrocardiogram tracing may show T wave changes, low voltage QRS complexes, shortened P–R intervals, prominent Q waves in V_5 and V_6, or bundle-branch block patterns (Fig.106).

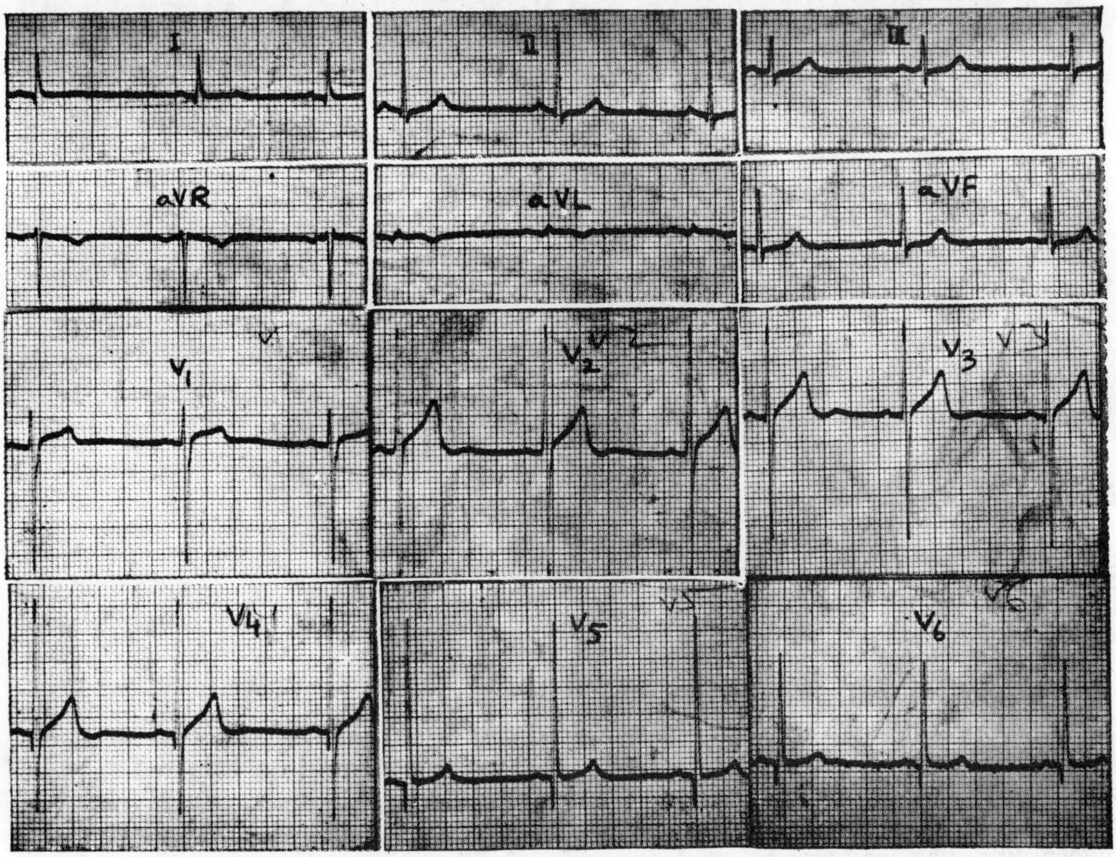

Fig. 106.
Fig.106 is an electrocardiogram from a case of pseudohypertrophic muscular dystrophy.

Dystrophia Myotonica

There may be T wave changes, bundle-branch block patterns or arrhythmias specially of supraventricular type.

Cerebral Vascular Accidents

The electrocardiogram may show a widened and prominent T wave which is usually inverted, and may be continuous with a large U wave (drawn out T–U complex); this is usually seen in the precordial leads. The Q–Tc interval may be prolonged; in some cases there may be slight depression of the S–T segment. Rarely a pattern of posterior myocardial infarction may be seen in the electrocardiogram (Figs. 107 & 108).

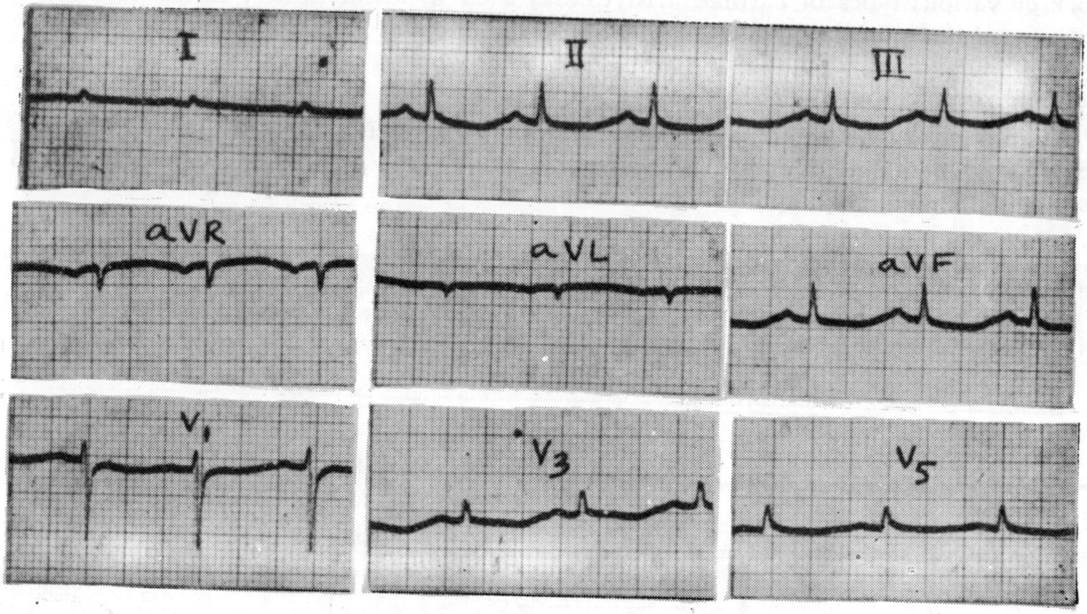

Fig. 107.

Fig. 107 shows an electrocardiogram from a male patient aged 53 years who had subarachnoid haemorrhage. The patient died after 6 days of the cerebral vascular accident.

Diphtheria

In diphtheria there may be atrial fibrillation or heart block; non-specific myocardial changes in the form of T wave changes may be seen. A depression of the S–T segment or a primary inversion of the T wave in a case of diphtheria is said to be characteristic of diphtheritic myocarditis.

Acute infections

In acute infections such as pneumonias, diphtheria, meningococcal septicaemia, acute tonsillitis, common cold, typhoid fever, mumps, poliomyelitis, bacterial endocarditis, scrub typhus, etc., characteristic changes in the electrocardiogram may be found as a result of peripheral circulatory failure, deficiency of B group of vitamins, and toxic myocarditis. This may give rise to degeneration, infiltration, exudate, necrosis and diffuse fibrosis of the myocardium; thus there may be arrhythmias including atrial flutter, atrial fibrillation, paroxysmal tachycardias, etc., P wave changes, conduction defects, depression of the S–T segment and T wave changes.

Parasitic infestations

Parasitic myocarditis following Chagas' disease may show evidence of right bundle-

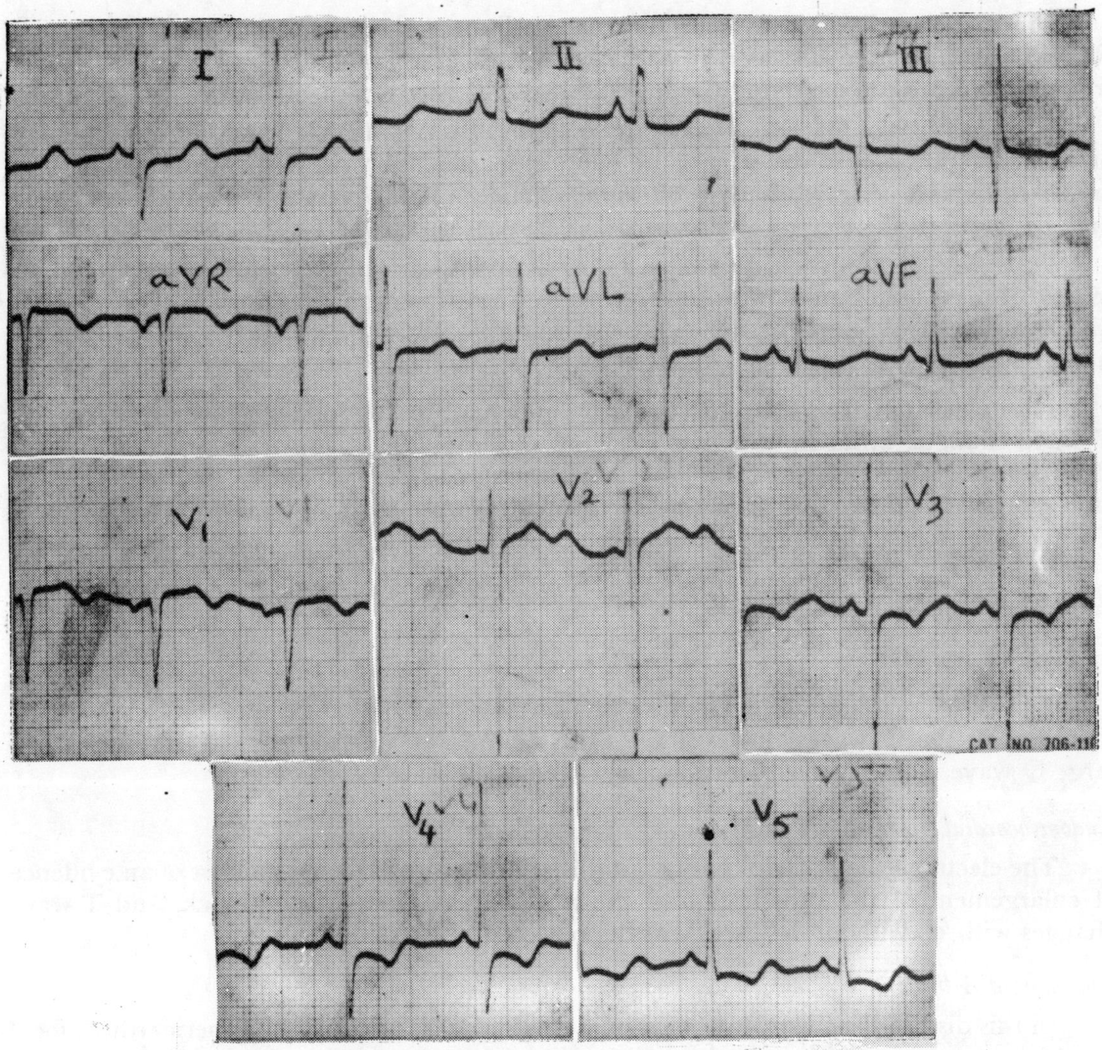

Fig.108.

Fig.108 shows an electrocardiogram from a male patient aged 66 years who had cerebral thrombosis of right cerebral hemisphere. The tracing became normal after one month.

branch block, often with left axis deviation, arrhythmias, heart block, etc., in the electrocardiogram.

Congenital or acquired toxoplasmosis may give evidence of myocarditis in the electrocardiogram ; transient myocardial ischaemic episodes may occur.

Myocarditis following trichiniasis may be found very rarely and there may be a prolonged P–R interval or S–A block and flat or inverted T waves in the electrocardiogram tracing on rare occasions.

Pulmonary schistosomiasis causing pulmonary endarteritis obliterans, may give rise to pulmonary hypertension and cor pulmonale; thus in the electrocardiogram there may be evidence of enlargement of right atrium and right ventricle with or without right ventricular strain.

Presence of a hydatid cyst in the myocardium and pericardium may show small R waves and inverted T waves in the electrocardiogram in unipolar chest leads taken from the precordium overlying the hydatid cyst.

Various types of filariasis such as those caused by Wuchereria bancrofti or W. malayi or onchocerciasis or Loa loa may cause endomyocardial fibrosis, right ventricular failure, endocarditis and pericarditis with effusion; changes characteristic of these abnormalities may be found in the electrocardiogram.

Pericarditis and myocarditis may follow actinomycosis of the heart; changes characteristic of these lesions may be found in the electrocardiographic tracing.

Coccidioido-mycotic infection may involve the myocardium and T wave changes in the electrocardiogram may be observed.

Histoplasma myocarditis and vegetative endocarditis due to Histoplasmosis may show T wave changes, atrial flutter, and evidence of individual chamber enlargement in the electrocardiographic tracing. In some cases there may be pericarditis with effusion and later constrictive pericarditis and the electrocardiogram may show S–T segment elevation, T wave inversion, atrial fibrillation or flutter, etc.

Cryptococcosis of the heart may show paroxysmal tachycardias and cardiac enlargement in the electrocardiogram.

Fiedler's Myocarditis

The electrocardiogram in Fiedler's myocarditis may show left bundle-branch block, inversion of the T waves, low voltage QRS complexes and occasionally there may be large Q wave with T wave inversion suggestive of myocardial infarction.

Endomyocardial Fibrosis

The electrocardiographic changes in this relatively rare disease, consist of an evidence of enlargement of the ventricles and the atria, arrhythmias, heart block, and T wave changes with or without S–T segment depression.

Rheumatoid Arthritis

In this disease the electrocardiographic tracing characteristic of the pericarditis, focal granulomatous myocarditis and cardiac chamber enlargement due to chronic valve lesions may be present.

Polyarteritis Nodosa

This condition may cause myocardial infarction due to involvement of the coronary artery and therefore evidence of myocardial infarction, myocardial ischaemia, ischaemic myocardial changes, arrhythmias, etc., may be found in the electrocardiographic tracing.

Systemic Lupus Erythematosus

The electrocardiogram may show an evidence of pericarditis, myocarditis and an evidence of enlargement of different chambers of the heart; the latter is due to verrucous endocarditis of the mitral, tricuspid or aortic valves.

Scleroderma Heart Disease

In systemic sclerosis, the first involvement of the heart is indicated by the presence of abnormality in the electrocardiographic tracing; there may be various types of conduction defects such as prolonged P–R interval, complete heart block, bundle-branch block, etc.; there may also be ectopic beats, other types of arrhythmias, ventricular hypertrophy or evidence of ischaemic heart disease, myocardial changes and evidence of cor pulmonale in the electrocardiogram (Fig. 109).

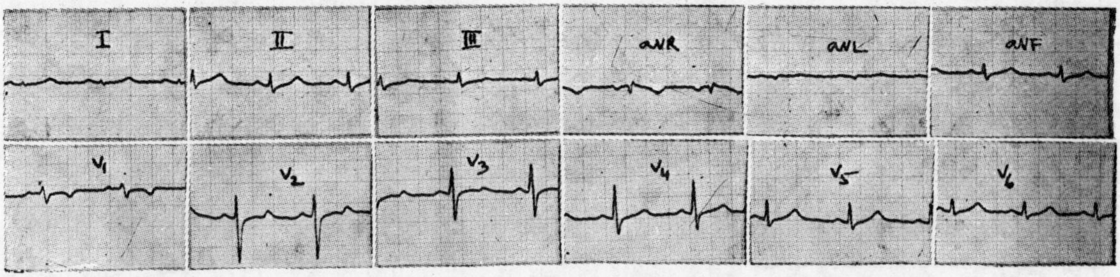

Fig. 109.

Fig. 109 shows an electrocardiogram from a case of scleroderma. There are low voltage QRS complexes and right ventricular strain.

Primary Amyloidosis

When the heart is involved the electrocardiogram may show low voltage complexes with prominent Q waves or QS patterns and inverted T waves.

Diabetes Mellitus

The electrocardiogram tracing may show S–T segment depression and T wave inversion probably due to a low serum potassium level especially after treatment of diabetic coma; these changes may also develop after hypoglycaemia following treatment with insulin; peripheral circulatory failure which may develop after diabetic coma may also produce same type of changes in the electrocardiogram. Associated coronary arterial disease which is common in diabetes mellitus may show all types of changes obtained in coronary arterial disease.

Haemochromatosis

In haemochromatosis the electrocardiogram may show S–T segment depression, T wave changes, cardiac arrhythmias including ventricular fibrillation and various types of heart block.

Cardiomyopathy

An evidence of enlargement of all chambers of the heart may be present along with T wave changes in the electrocardiographic tracing; there may also be various types of cardiac arrhythmias; recurrent pulmonary embolism may cause pulmonary hypertension which may show evidence of cor pulmonale in the electrocardiographic tracing. Rarely there may be evidence of myocardial infarction (Fig. 110).

Acute Nephritis

In this case there is hypertension, retention of sodium, increased venous pressure and inflammation of the capillaries of toxic or allergic origin; in the electrocardiogram there may thus be an evidence of enlargement of all the chambers of the heart, S–T segment depression and inversion of the T wave.

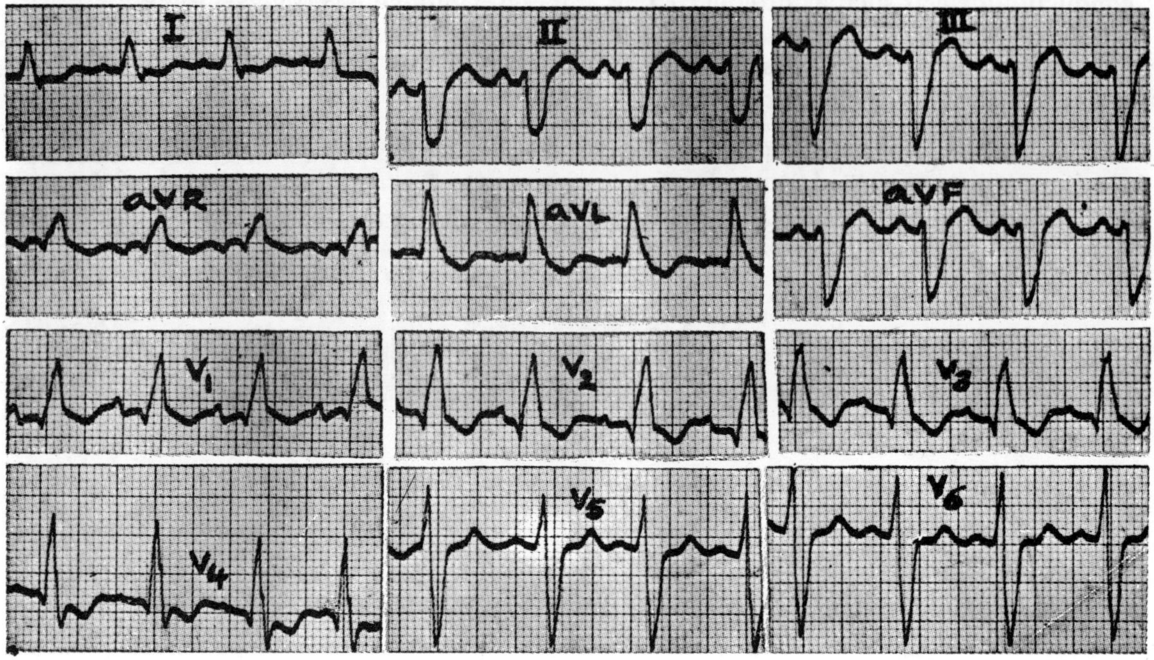

Fig.110.

Fig. 110 is an electrocardiogram from a case of cardiomyopathy showing intraventricular conduction defect.

Uraemia

The changes in the electrocardiogram in uraemia is due to a high level of serum potassium; thus there may be tall, sharp and high voltage T waves. Inverted T waves due to any cause other than that due to myocardial infarction may be corrected with the onset of uraemia with a high serum potassium level. The P waves and the QRS complexes may be widened.

Primary Neoplasm of the Heart

In the left atrial myxoma there may be atrial fibrillation, some enlargement of left atrium and right ventricle.

In right atrial primary sarcoma or haemangioendotheliosarcoma an evidence of right atrial enlargement may be present in the electrocardiogram.

In fibroma of the left ventricle there may be paroxysmal ventricular tachycardia and a pattern suggestive of myocardial infarction in the left ventricular surface leads may be present.

Single or multiple rhabdomyomata chiefly involving the left ventricle may show cardiac arrhythmias, prominent Q waves, S–T segment and T wave changes in the electrocardiogram.

Secondary Neoplasm of the Heart

Secondary neoplasm of the heart from bronchogenic carcinoma, breast carcinoma, thymic or other mediastinal tumours, etc., may involve the pericardium and other parts of the heart giving rise to atrial flutter, fibrillation or paroxysmal atrial tachycardia, S–T segment changes, T wave changes and heart block in the electrocardiogram.

Leukaemia

In leukaemia the electrocardiogram may show S–T segment elevation and T wave changes due to pericarditis, T wave changes and cardiac arrhythmias due to myocardial infiltration, S–T segment depression due to myocardial ischaemia and prominent Q wave, S–T segment elevation and T wave inversion due to coronary thrombosis in elderly persons; associated severe anaemia may show evidence of hyperkinetic circulatory state.

Carcinoid Disease

In carcinoid disease of the small intestine there may be stenosis at the pulmonary and tricuspid valve levels with an evidence of enlargement of the right ventricle and right atrium respectively.

Toxaemias of Pregnancy

In these cases there may be inversion of the T wave in leads V_4 to V_6 and sometimes evidence of ventricular enlargement.

Effects of Radiation on the Heart

Abnormal elevation or depression of the S–T segment and T wave changes may develop in the electrocardiogram due to myocardial damage caused by irradiation; these changes are usually seen about 4 months after irradiation and may take about a year to disappear after cessation of irradiation treatment.

CHAPTER XVI

EFFECTS OF DRUGS ON THE ELECTROCARDIOGRAM

DIGITALIS

Different types of arrhythmias such as sinus bradycardia, premature or ectopic beats, paroxysmal atrial tachycardia with A–V block, nodal rhythm, partial or complete A–V block, atrial flutter, atrial fibrillation, paroxysmal nodal or ventricular tachycardia, ventricular bigeminy, ventricular fibrillation, etc., may develop following digitalis overdosage; low serum potassium level potentiates digitalis toxicity. A characteristic sagging depression of the RS–T segment with the T wave gradually absorbed in it, is usually seen in the leads V_4 to V_6 in left ventricular hypertrophy and in the leads V_1 and V_2 in right ventricular hypertrophy (Fig. 111); the sagging depression may also be well seen in the standard limb leads. The Q–T interval is shortened.

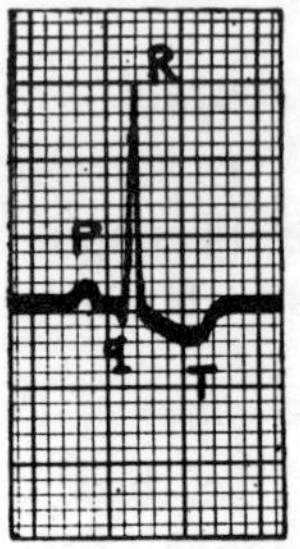

Fig. 111.

Fig. 111 is a diagrammatic representation of changes in S–T segment and T waves after digitalis overdosage.

EMETINE

A condition of toxic myocarditis may develop after intramuscular injection of emetine hydrochloride and the electrocardiographic tracing may show T wave inversion and prolonged Q–T interval; occasionally there may be S–T depression, and prolonged P–R interval. The changes usually disappear after a few weeks of discontinuation of emetine therapy.

QUINIDINE

Quinidine possesses a vagolytic action and tends to accelerate the conduction of the excitatory impulses through the A–V node so that the P–R interval may be shortened. It may depress the S–T segment, flatten T wave and prolong Q–T interval (corrected); it may eliminate ectopic focus by depressing the myocardium. In atrial fibrillation of recent origin it may produce atrial flutter or atrial tachycardia and cause increased ventricular rate unless the patient is previously digitalised; when atrial fibrillation is old it may cause cardiac standstill. When large doses of quinidine are used it may produce various degrees of A–V block, A–V dissociation, nodal rhythm, idioventricular rhythm, ventricular tachycardia, cardiac standstill, and widening of the QRS complexes.

PROCAINAMIDE

Effects of procainamide on the heart are similar to those of quinidine but are of lesser degree. Its effects are, however, more on the ventricles than on the atria. Prolonged P–R intervals, prolonged Q–T intervals and widened QRS complexes are common. When used intravenously it may produce ventricular ectopic beats, widening of the QRS complexes and cardiogenic shock.

HYPERPOTASSAEMIA

Any condition giving rise to hyperpotassaemia especially aided by hyponatraemia may show various changes in stages in the electrocardiographic tracing. A tall and pointed T wave, depressed S–T segment, prolonged P–R interval, a low and wide P wave, intraventricular conduction defect, prolonged Q–T interval, ventricular arrhythmias, sinus bradycardia, ventricular flutter, atrial and ventricular asystole may all develop ultimately leading to cardiac standstill (Fig. 112).

HYPOPOTASSAEMIA

Hypopotassaemia from any cause may show a prolonged P–R interval, a depressed S–T segment, a low or inverted T wave and a prominent U wave, with a prolonged Q–T interval (Fig. 113).

HYPERCALCAEMIA

Hypercalcaemia may cause sinus arrhythmia, sinus bradycardia, ectopic beats, A–V heart block, wandering pacemaker and shortened Q–T interval in the electrocardiographic tracing.

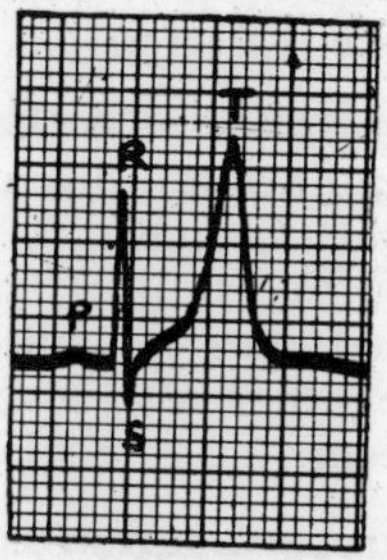

Fig. 112.

Fig. 112 is a diagrammatic representation of electrocardiogram in hyperpotassaemia.

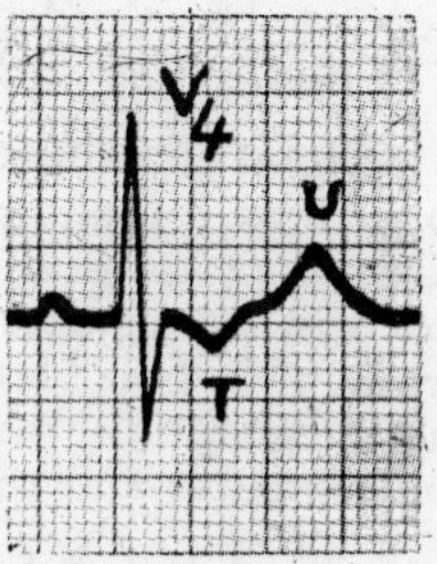

Fig. 113.

Fig. 113 is a diagrammatic representation of electrocardiogram in hypopotassaemia.

ADRENALINE

Adrenaline may induce any type of cardiac arrhythmias such as ectopic beats, paroxysmal tachycardia, flutter or fibrillation, inversion of the T waves specially in leads V_4 to V_6; existing coronary insufficiency may be aggravated further, causing further depression of the S–T segment.

ANAESTHETICS AND HYPOTHERMIA

Administration of anaesthetics such as chloroform may cause ventricular fibrillation and sudden death.

When hypothermia is used electrocardiogram may show various changes depending on the temperature maintained during the operative procedure. At about 30°C. bradycardia and prolonged Q–Tc interval may be found; at about 26°C. various types of arrhythmias of atrial origin or heart block may appear; at about 22°C. ventricular fibrillation or cardiac arrest may take place.

NICOTINE

Heavy smokers may absorb excessive nicotine and may show evidence of coronary insufficiency, atrial fibrillation and ectopic beats in the electrocardiographic tracing.

BARIUM CHLORIDE

Ingestion of barium chloride may cause ventricular fibrillation and ectopic beats.

PHENYLBUTAZONE

Administration of phenylbutazone may show evidence of ventricular enlargement. Cardiac arrhythmias such as atrial fibrillation and evidence of pericarditis may also be seen.

TARTAR EMETIC

In the treatment of schistosomiasis a full course of tartar emetic may cause a low, flat or inverted T wave, becoming normal after discontinuance of the therapy.

CHAPTER XVII

FOETAL ELECTROCARDIOGRAM AND ELECTROCARDIOGRAM IN INFANTS

Methods had been devised to record electrocardiograms of foetus in pregnant mothers. This cannot be recorded without simultaneous recording of the Ecg. of the mother and the heart rates of the mother and foetus are different.

A foetal electrocardiogram is taken with the help of a standard electrocardiograph machine equipped with a preamplifier capable of amplifying an input signal 50 times, recording being made in a frequency range of 12–20 cycles/second ; in this way both foetal and maternal ecg. may be recorded in a pregnant woman. The subject lies down after evacuation of her bladder. One electrode of bi-polar lead is placed over the abdomen in the mid-line at the level of the fundus of the pregnant uterus and the other lead over the abdomen in the midline just above the symphysis pubis and then the recording of ecg. is made.

A recording of foetal electrocardiogram is necessary for the following reasons :

(1) To confirm whether the foetus is alive or not, specially during the second and third trimesters of pregnancy.

(2) To detect cardiac arrhythmias in foetus.

(3) To diagnose multiple pregnancy in the early stage.

(4) To monitor foetal heart rate during labour.

(5) To determine the position of the foetus inside the uterus.

When the mother's QRS vector is normal, that is, inferiorly directed, QRS complexes are upright ; in such a situation the foetal QRS complexes in a vertex presentation would be downwards because of the upward direction of the foetal cardiac vector (vide fig. 114).

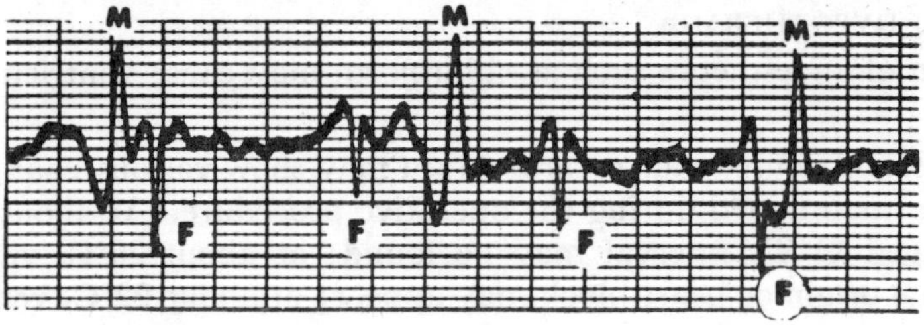

Fig. 114

Fig. 114 The above Ecg. tracing is that a foetus with vertex presentation; the maternal QRS complexes (marked 'M') are in an upward direction whereas the foetal QRS complexes (marked as 'F') are in a downward direction.

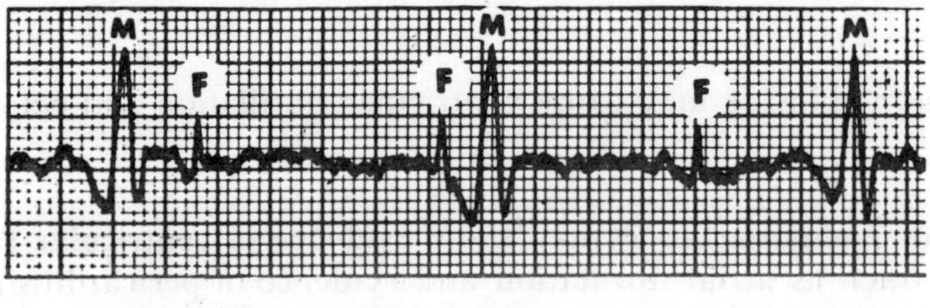

Fig. 115

Fig. 115 The above Ecg. tracing shows that of a foetus with a breech presentation showing maternal QRS complexes (marked 'M') in an upward direction and the foetal QRS complexes (marked 'F') are also in the upward direction i.e. in the same direction as those of the mother.

In a breech presentation of the foetus with mother's QRS vector being normal, foetal cardiac vector would be directed inferiorly ; this would produce foetal QRS complexes upright (vide fig. 115). Thus the foetal electrocardiogram would help to ascertain the position of the foetus in the uterus of the mother which would help to decide proper steps to be taken before delivery.

Electrocardiograms in infants and children.

In foetus right ventricle works more compared to the left ventride. Therefore at birth and in infants there would be right ventricular dominance with or without right ventricular strain indicated by a tall R wave in V_1 lead and a symmetrical inversion of T wave in V_1 to V_3 leads (vide fig. 116). There would also be right axis deviation as judged from the standard bipolar limb leads-I and III. There would also be a vertical lie i.e. a vertical heart position known from a tall R in aVR and a deep S wave in aVL lead (vide fig. 117).

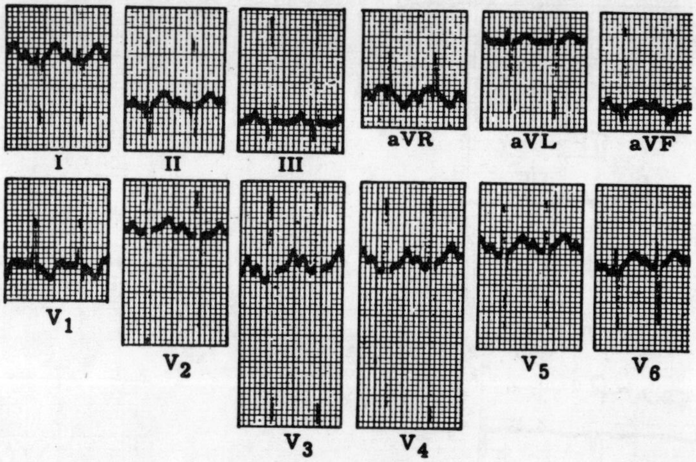

Fig. 116

Fig. 116 The above Ecg. tracing is that of an infant 2 days old. There is right axis, vertical lie (tall R in aVR and deep S in aVL) and right ventricular dominance (a tall R in V_1 lead).

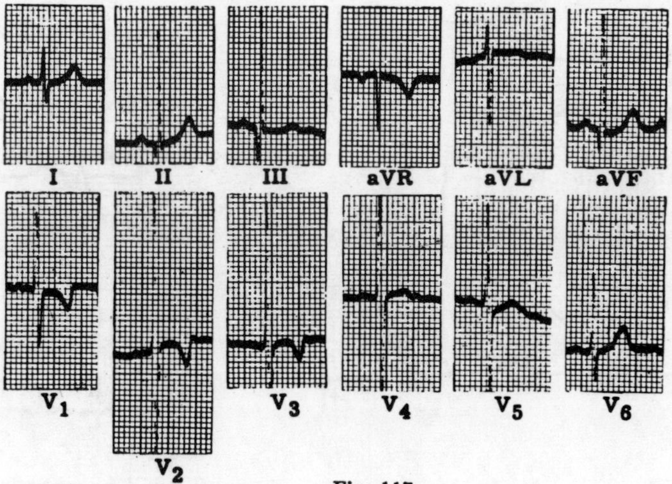

Fig. 117

Fig. 117 The above Ecg. tracing shows a normal Ecg. in a 9 yr. old child. There is vertical lie (deep S in aVL, tall R wave in V_1 and inverted T wave S in V_{1-3})

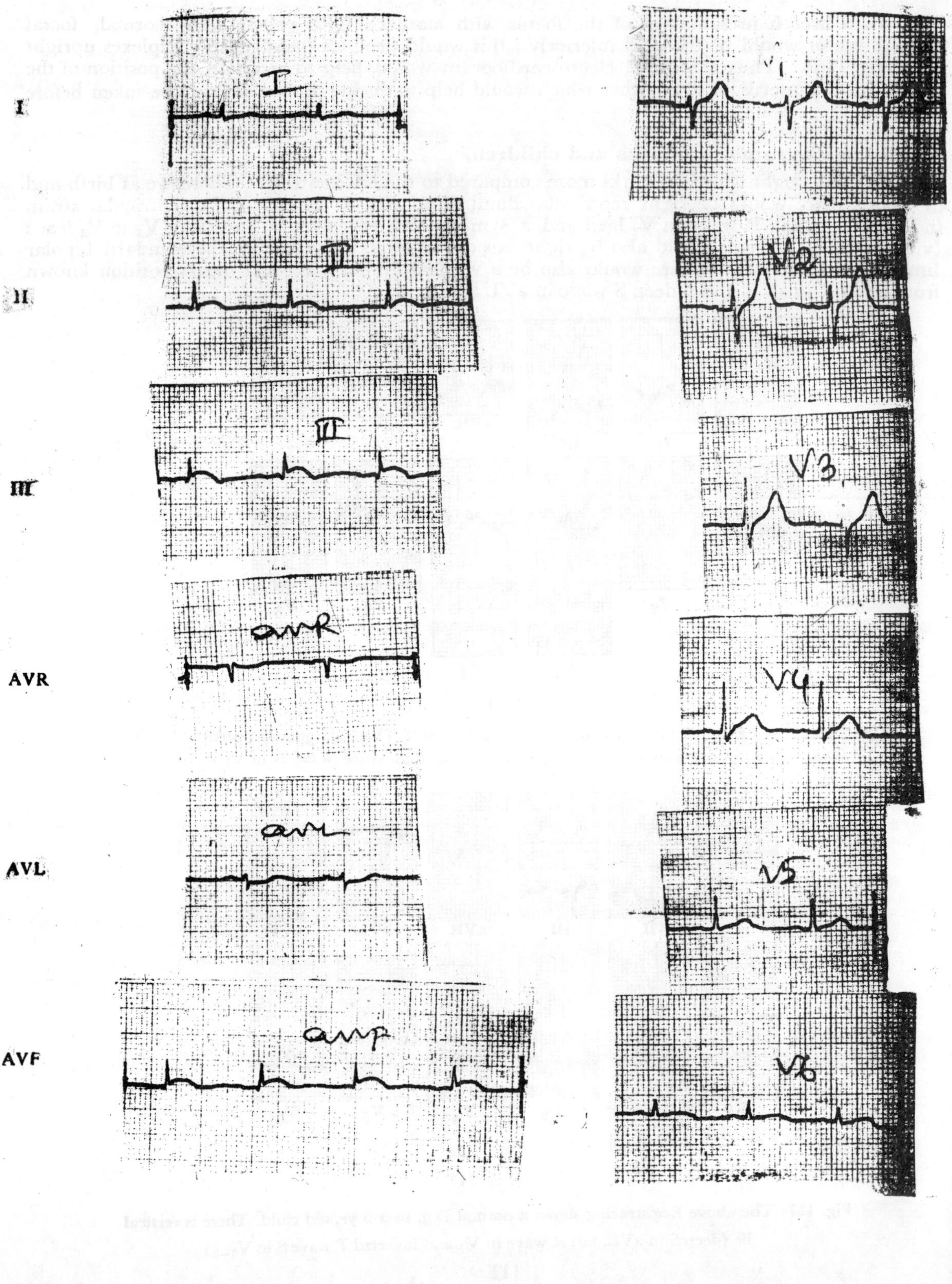
I
II
III
AVR
AVL
AVF

CHAPTER XVIII

REVIEW TRACINGS

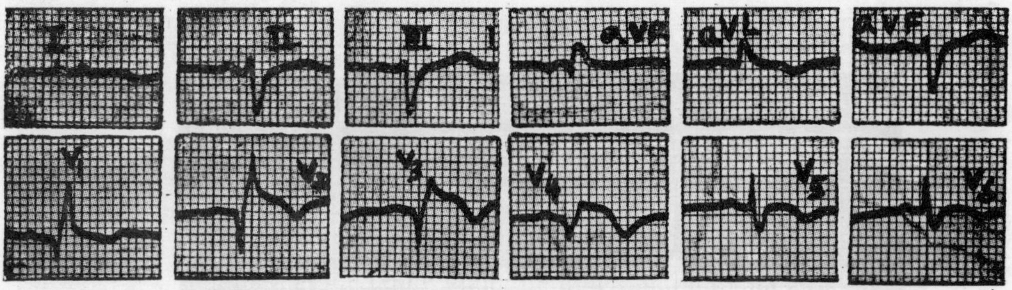

Review Tracing 1.*

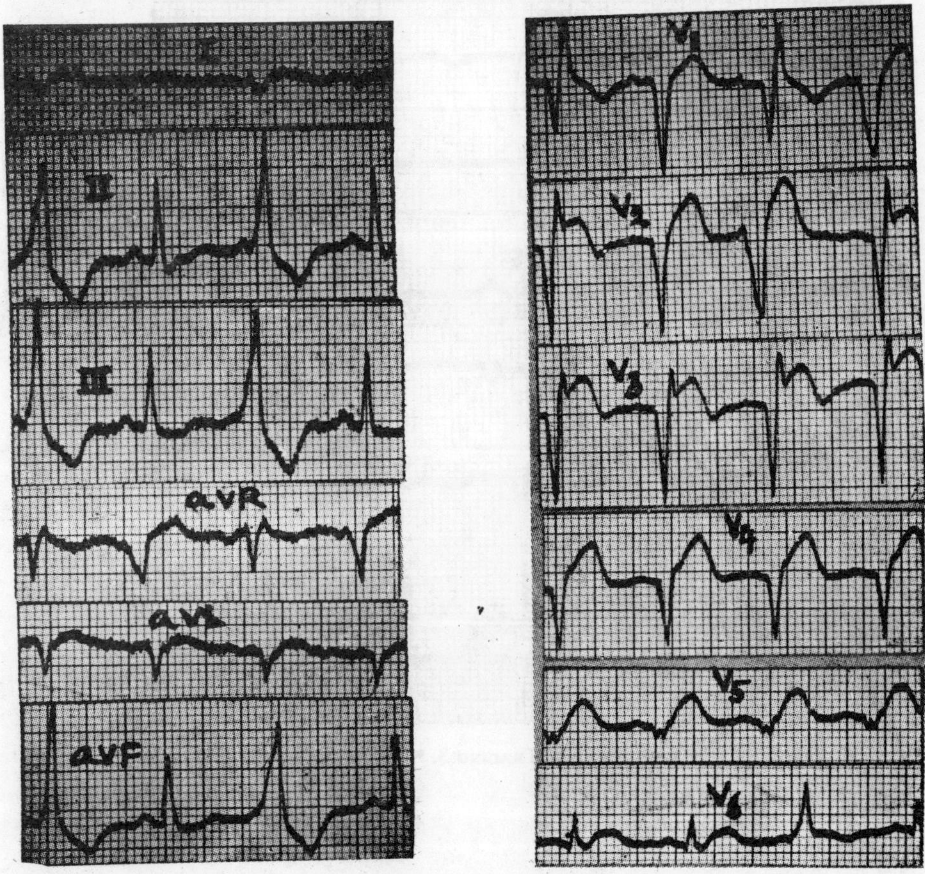

Review Tracing 2.*

* For interpretation *vide* page 154

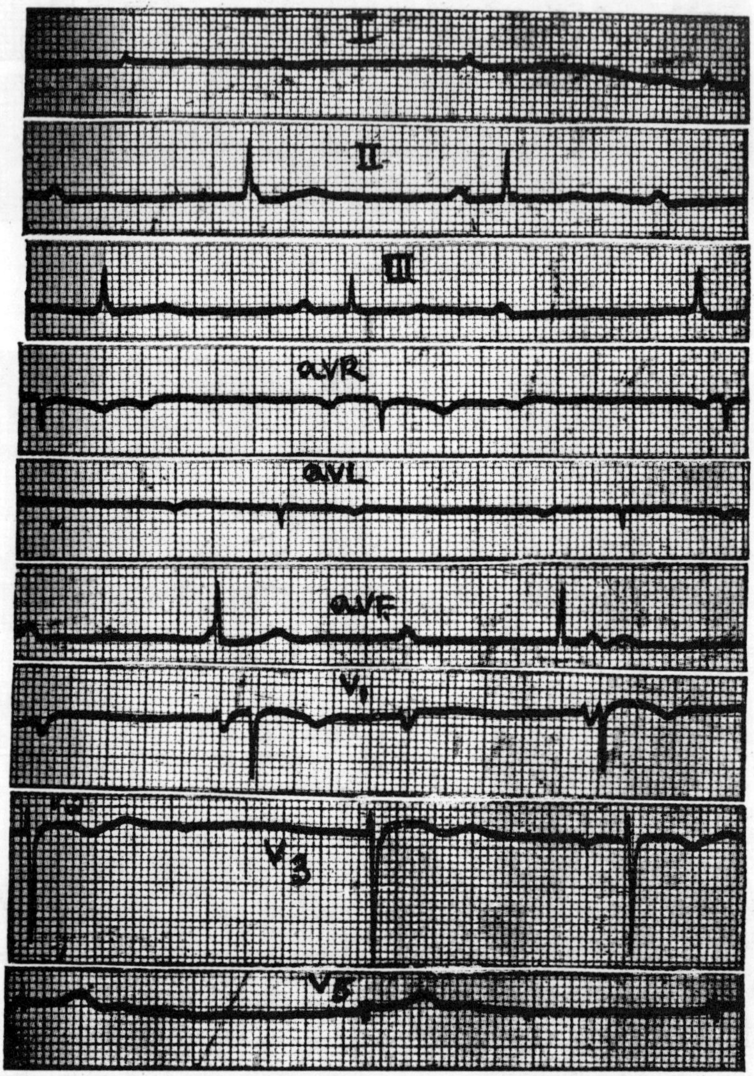

REVIEW TRACING 3. *

* For interpretation *vide* page 154

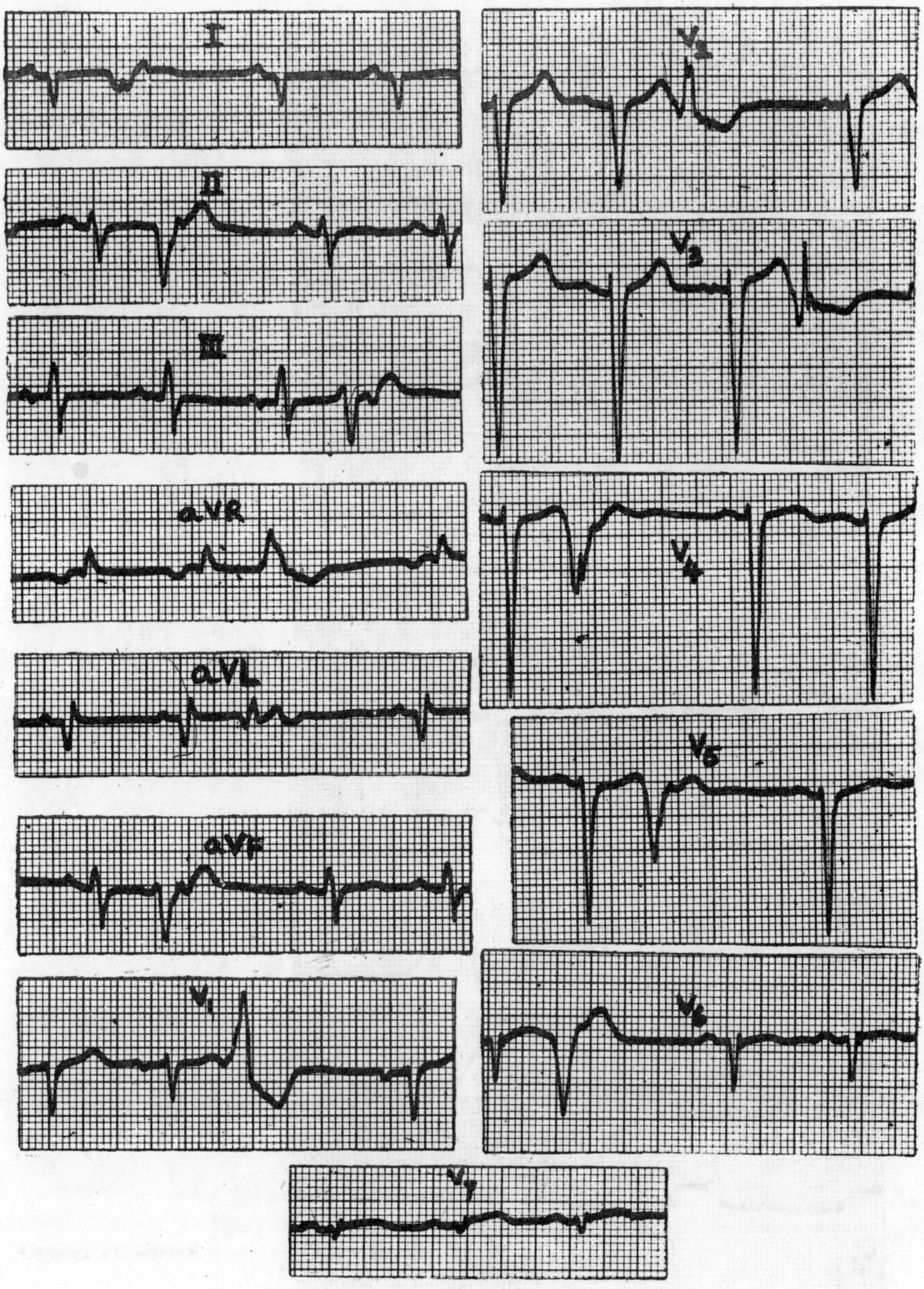

REVIEW TRACING 4.*

* For interpretation *vide* page 154

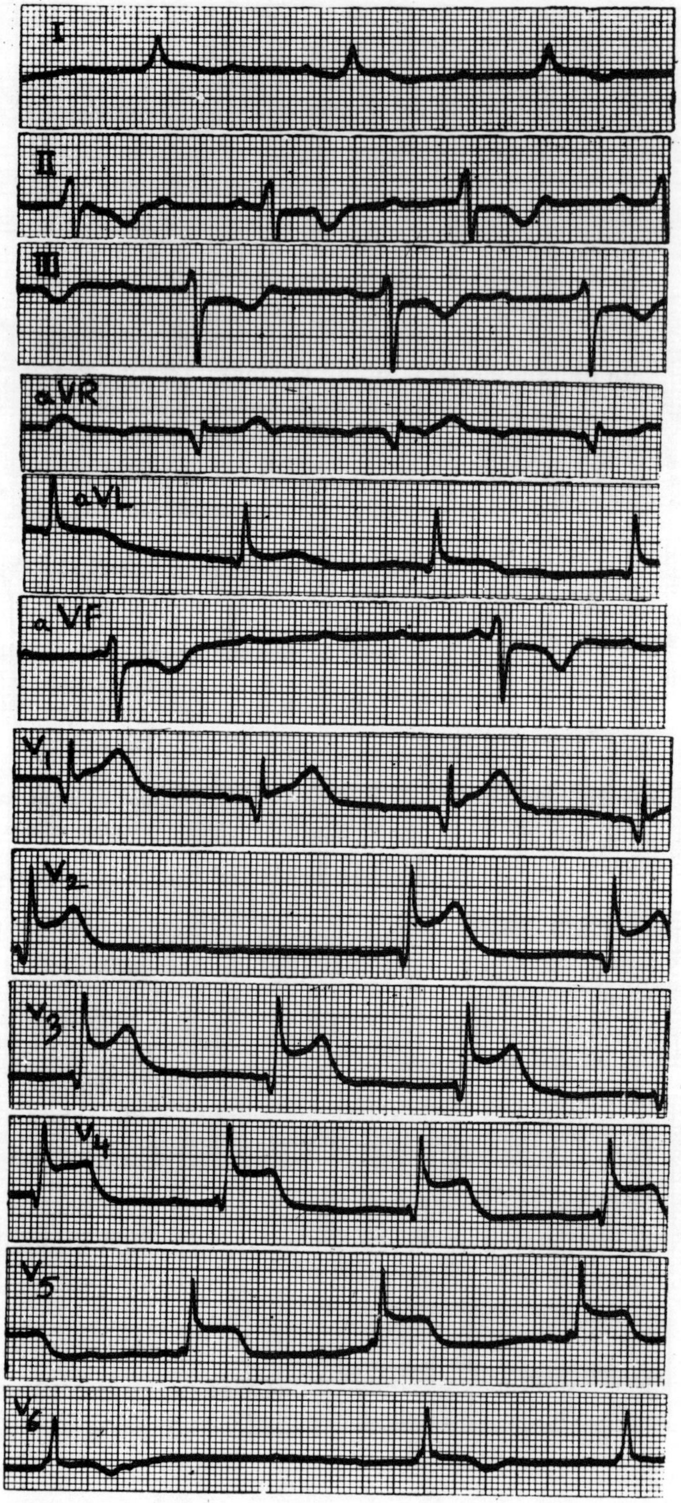

REVIEW TRACING 5.*

* For interpretation *vide* page 154

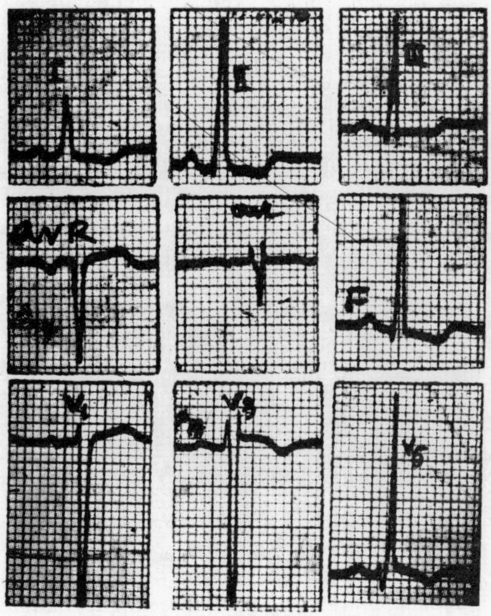

REVIEW TRACING 6.*

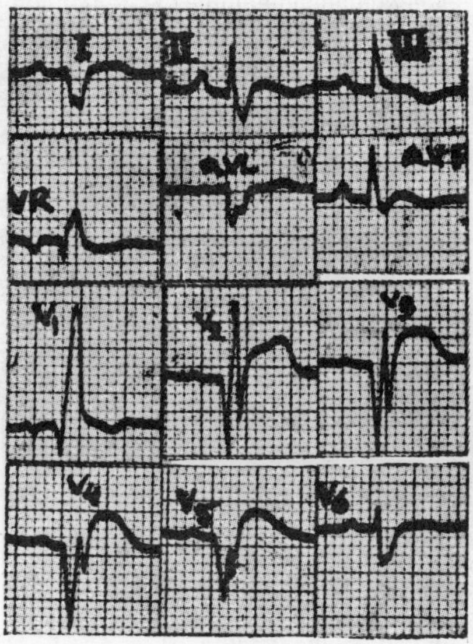

REVIEW TRACING 7.*

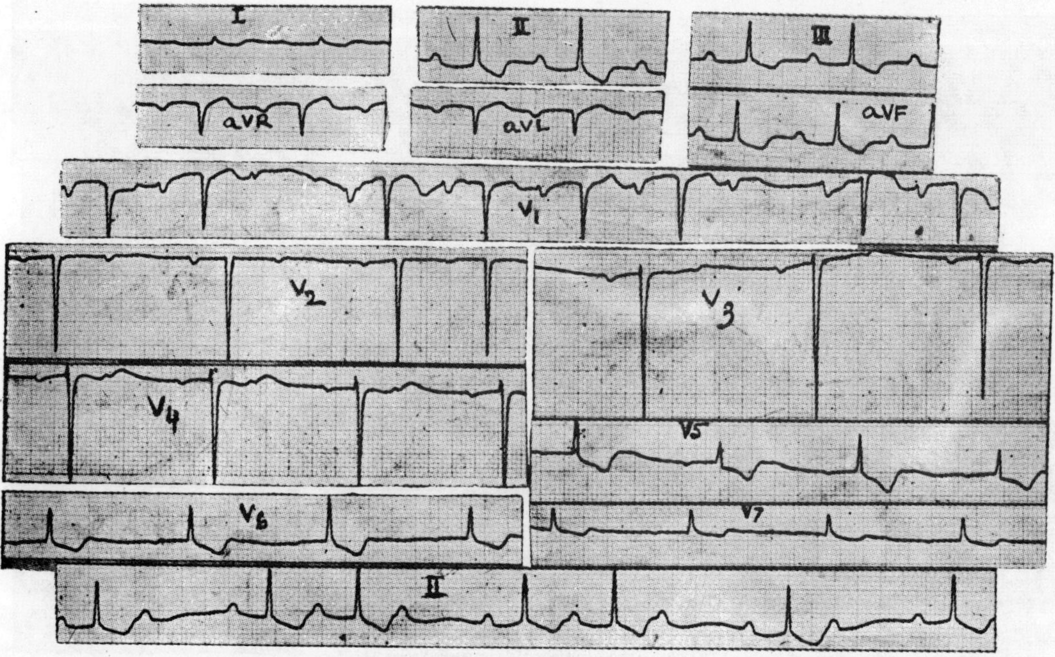

REVIEW TRACING 8.*

* For interpretation *vide* page 154

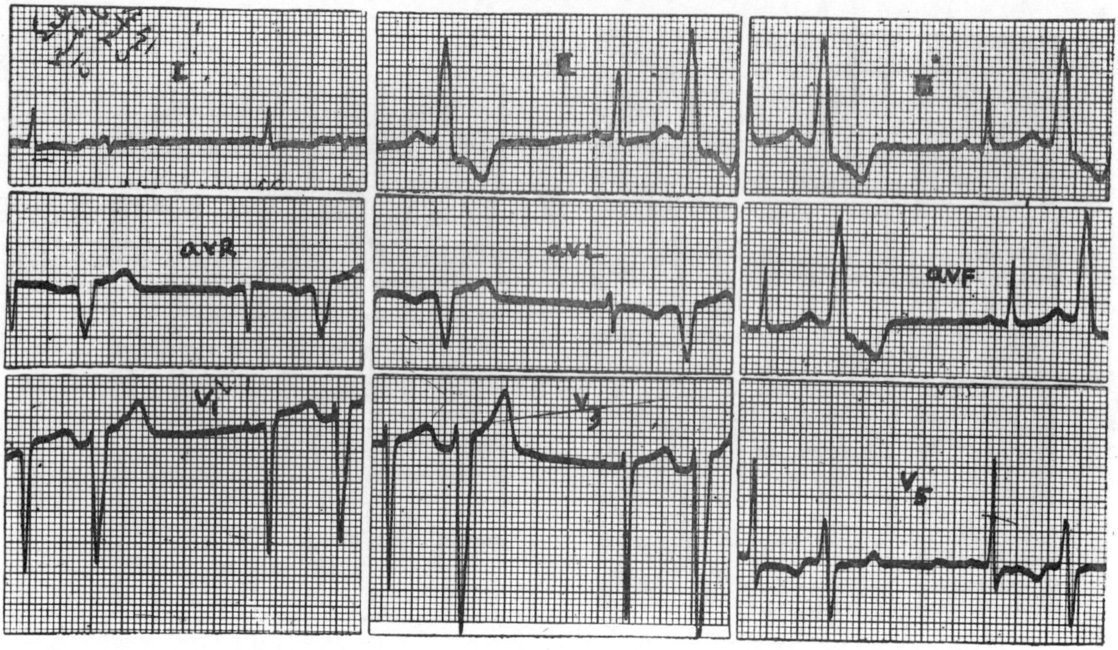

REVIEW TRACING 9.*

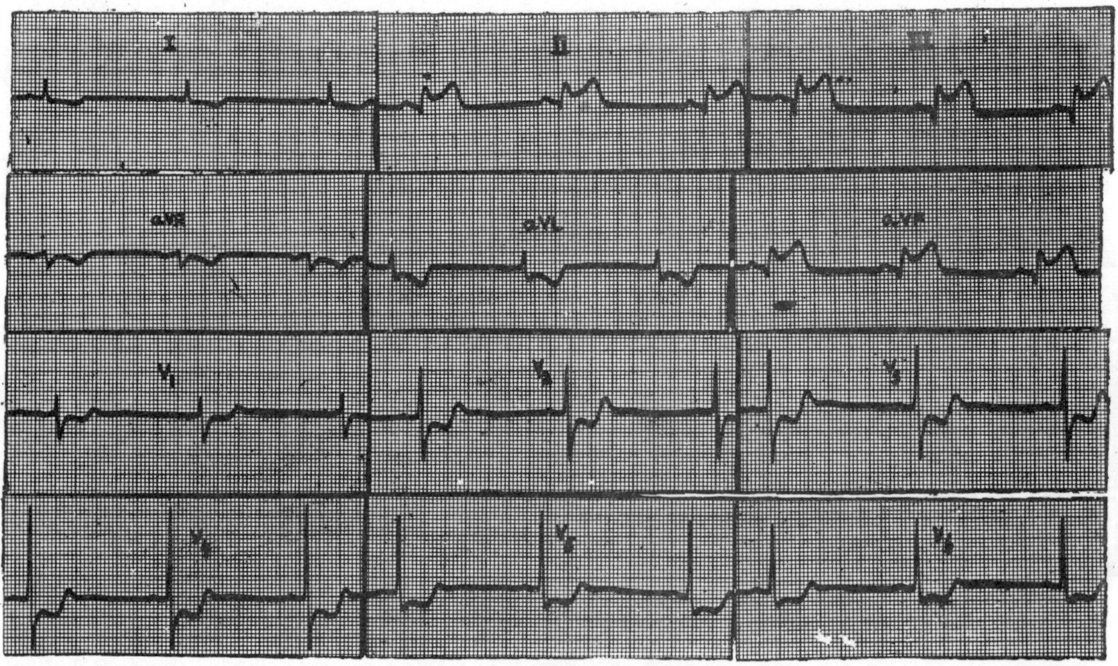

REVIEW TRACING 10.*

* For interpretation *vide* page 154

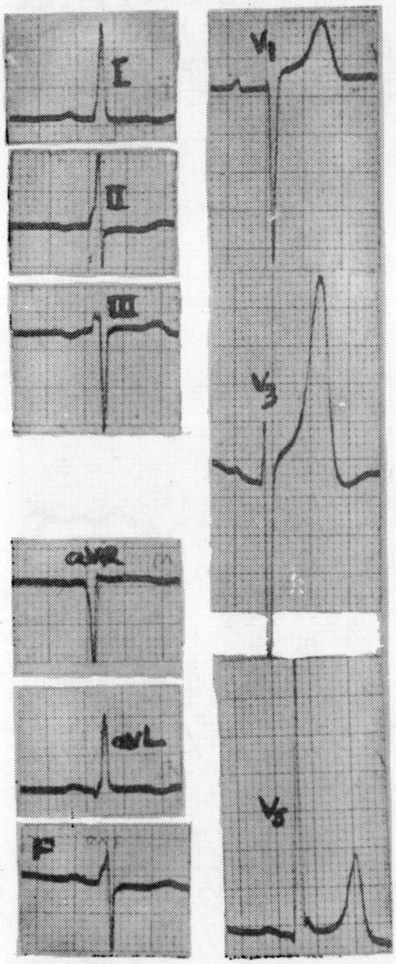

Review Tracing 11.*

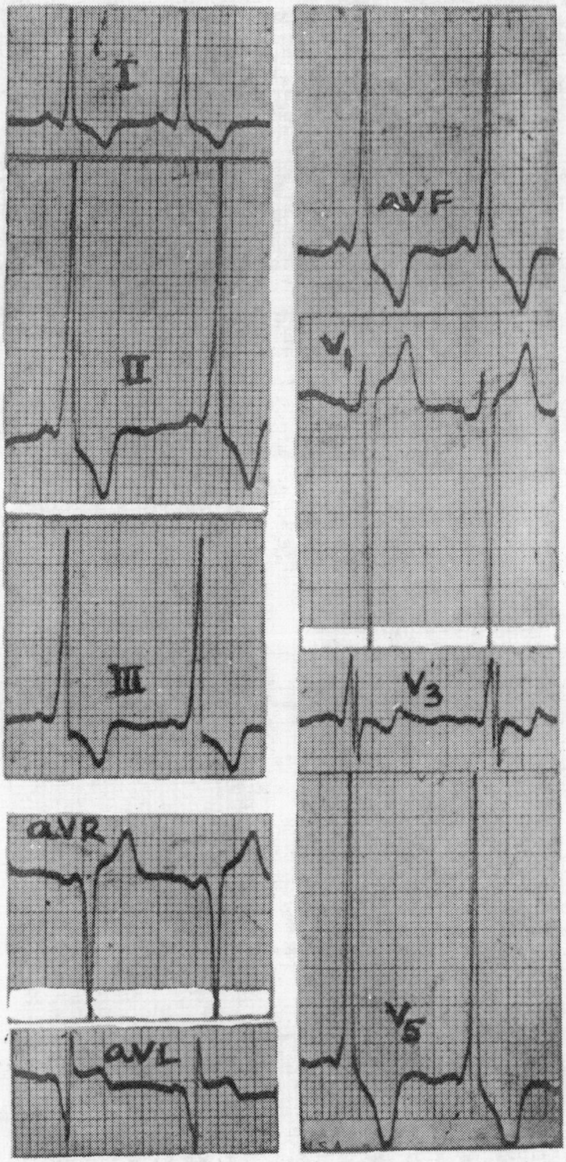

Review Tracing 12.*

*For interpretation *vide* page 154

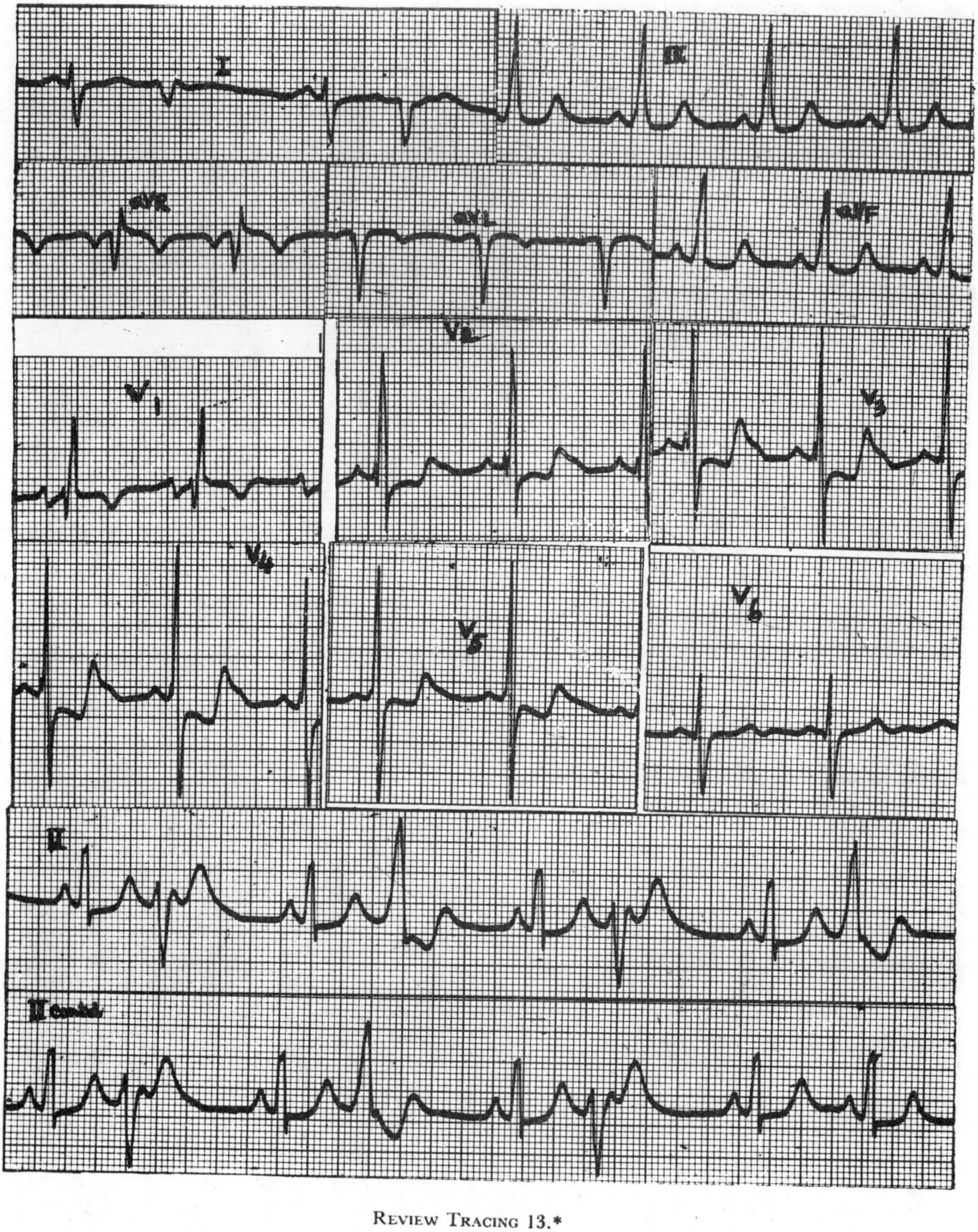

REVIEW TRACING 13.*

*For interpretation *vide* page 154

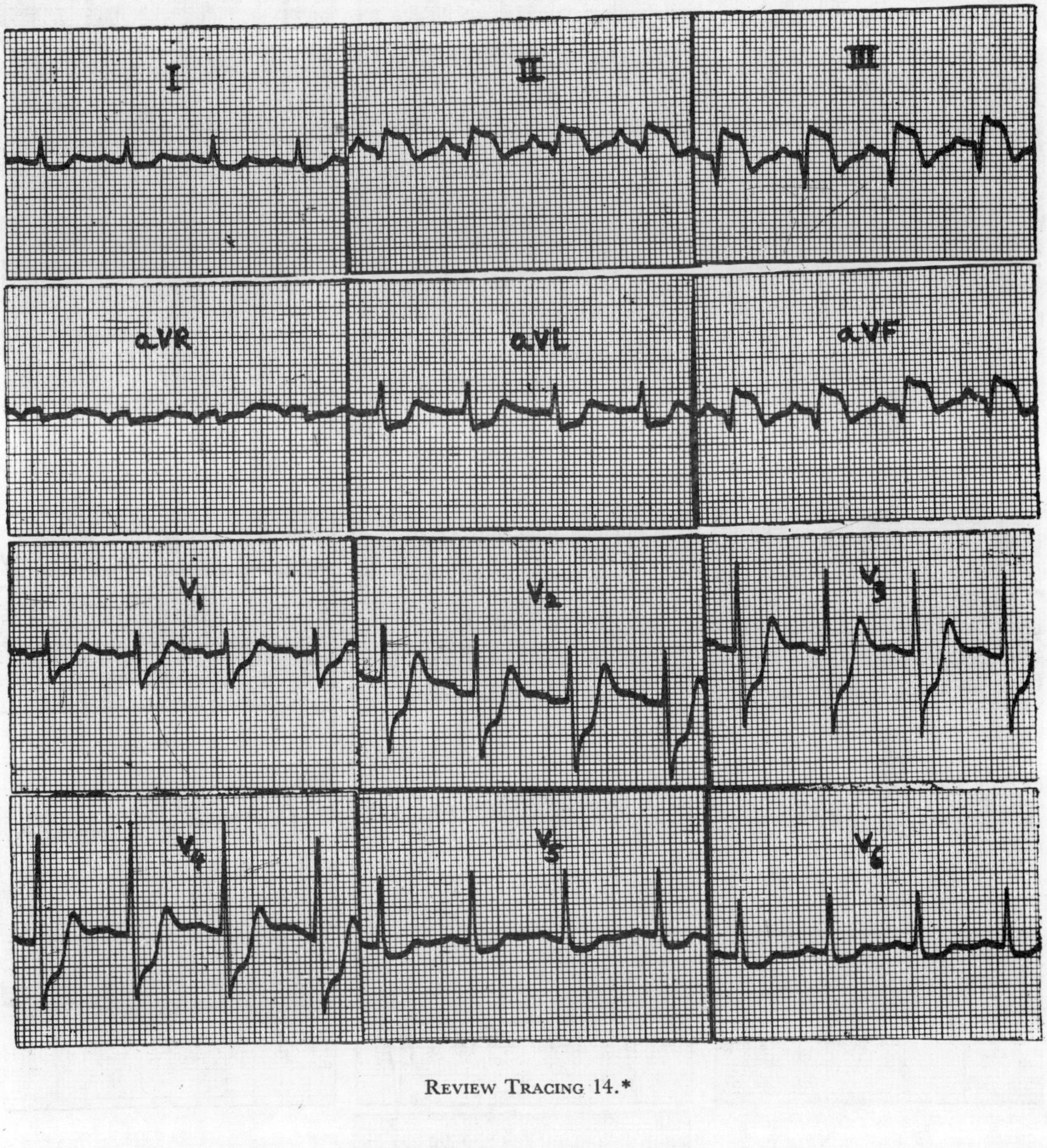

REVIEW TRACING 14.*

* For interpretation *vide* page 154

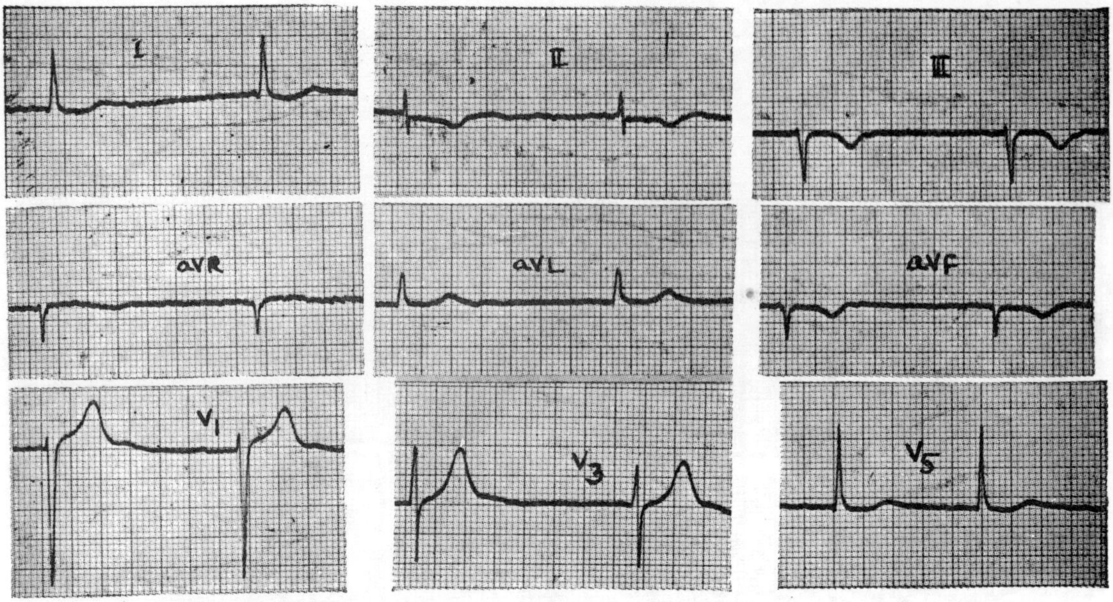

REVIEW TRACING 15.*

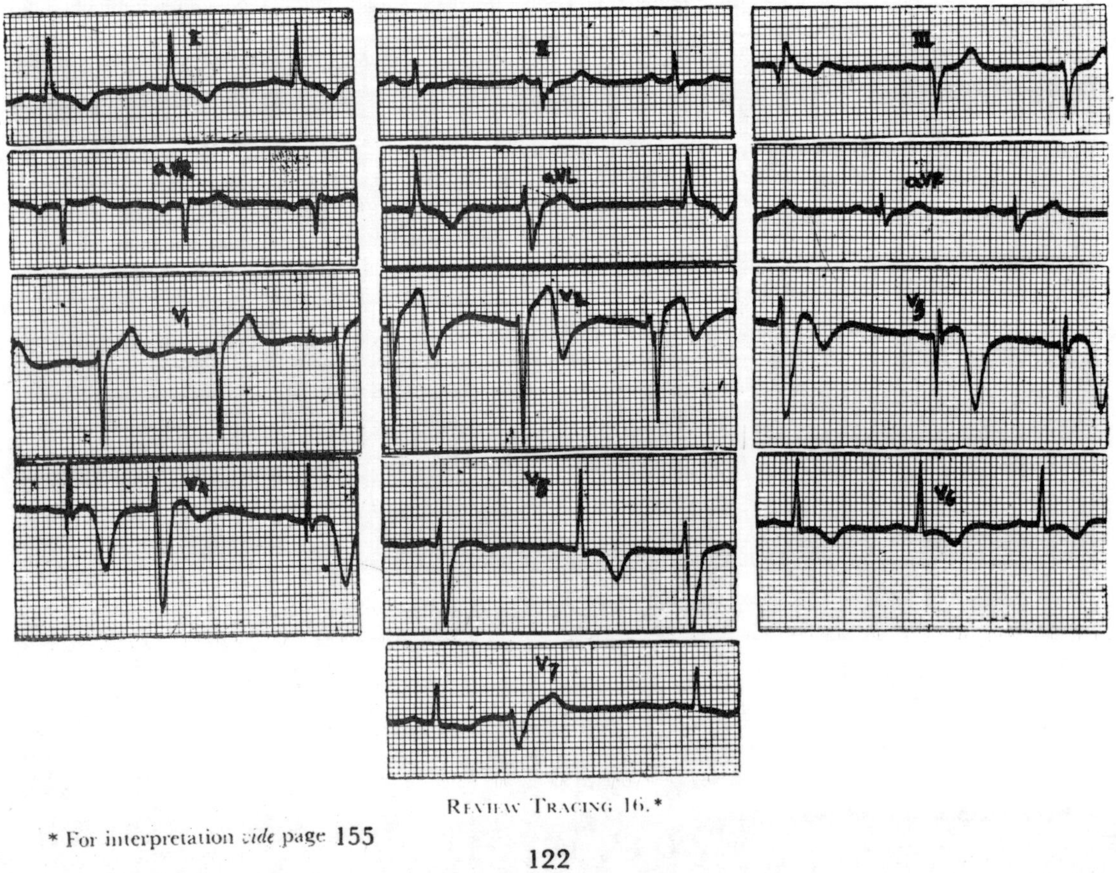

REVIEW TRACING 16.*

* For interpretation *vide* page 155

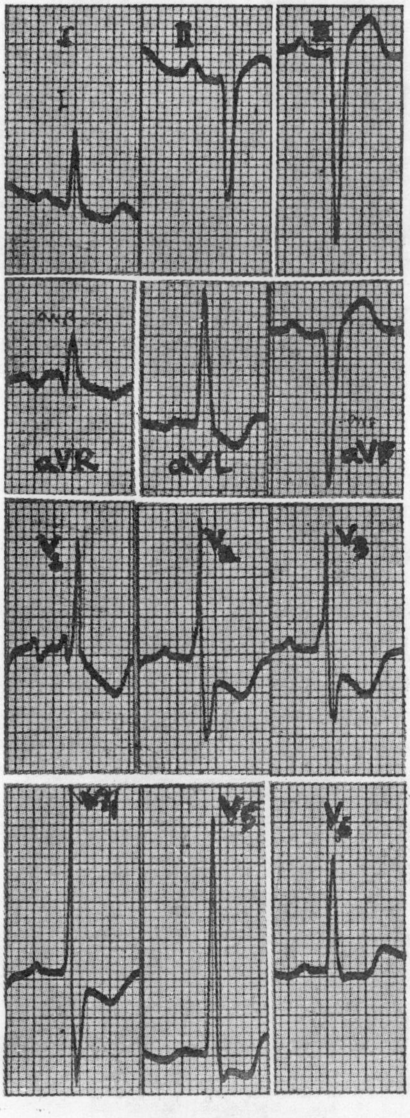

REVIEW TRACING 17.*

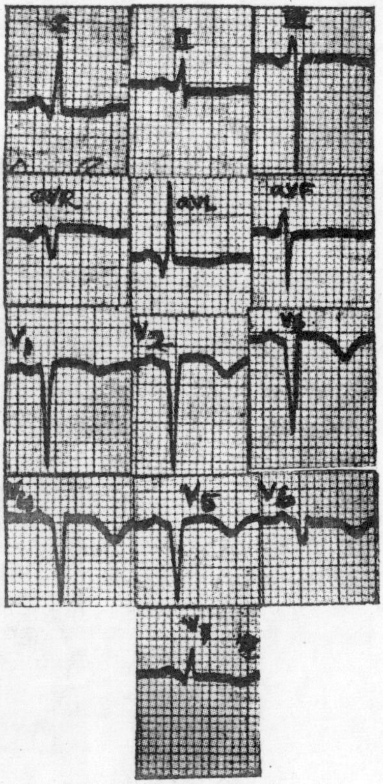

REVIEW TRACING 18.*

*For interpretation *vide* page 155

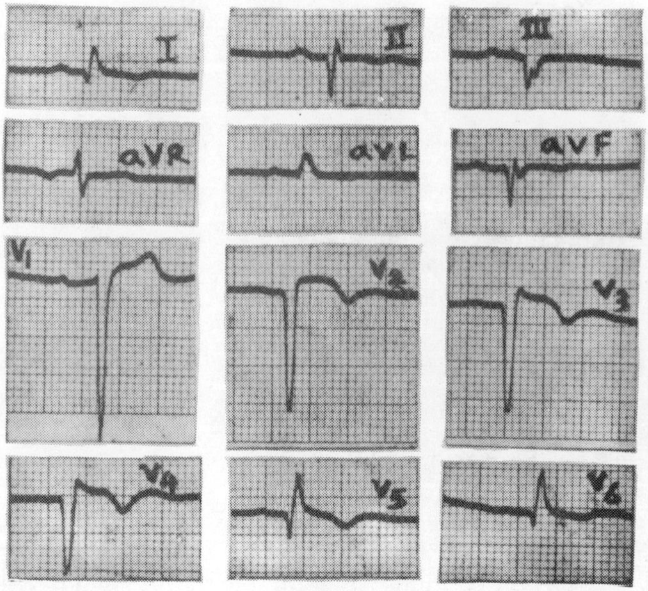

REVIEW TRACING 19.*

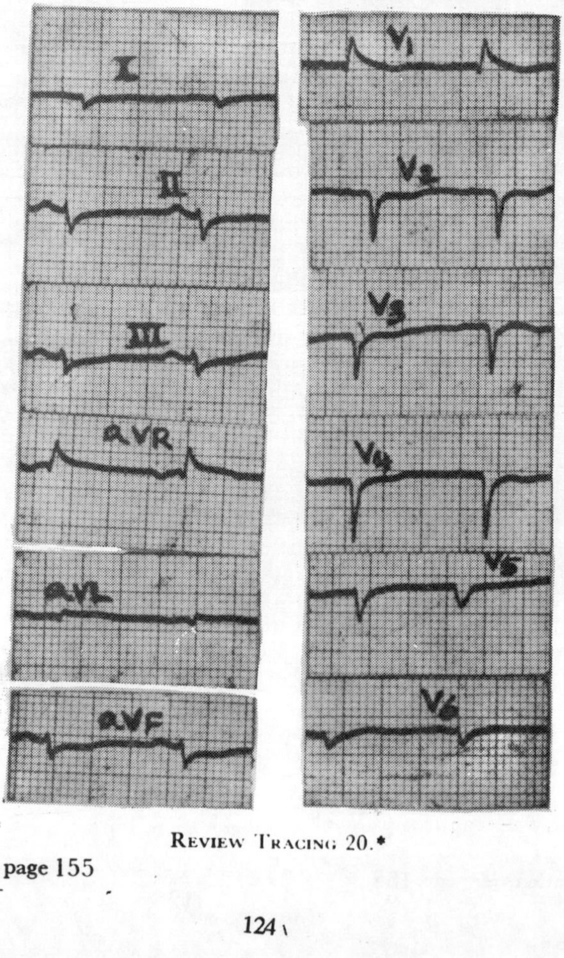

REVIEW TRACING 20.*

* For interpretation *vide* page 155

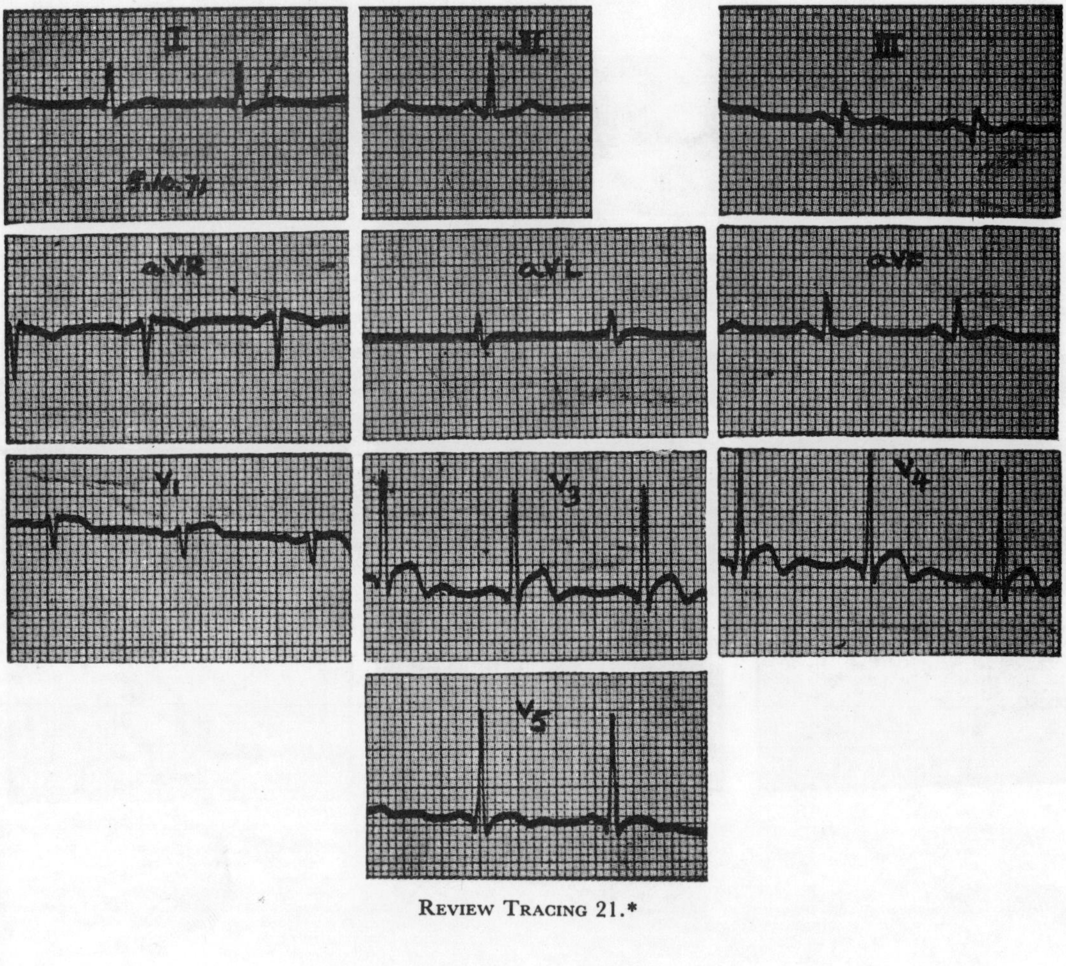

REVIEW TRACING 21.*

* For interpretation *vide* page 155

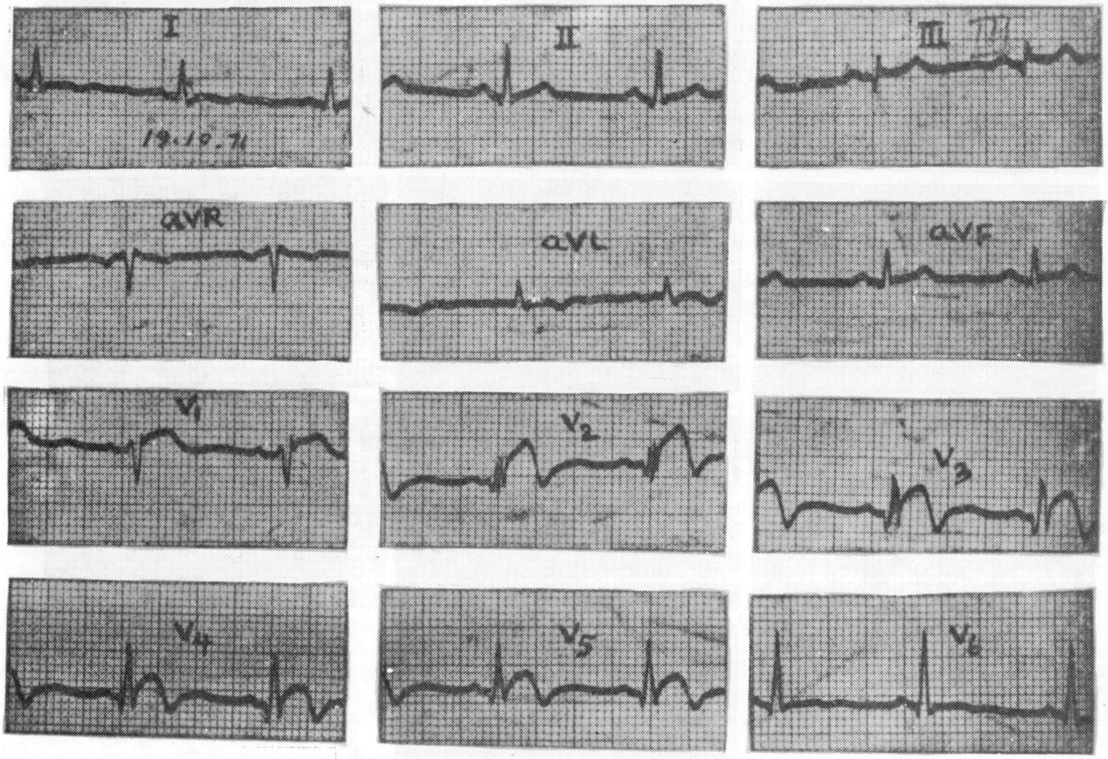

REVIEW TRACING 22.*

* For interpretation *vide* page 155

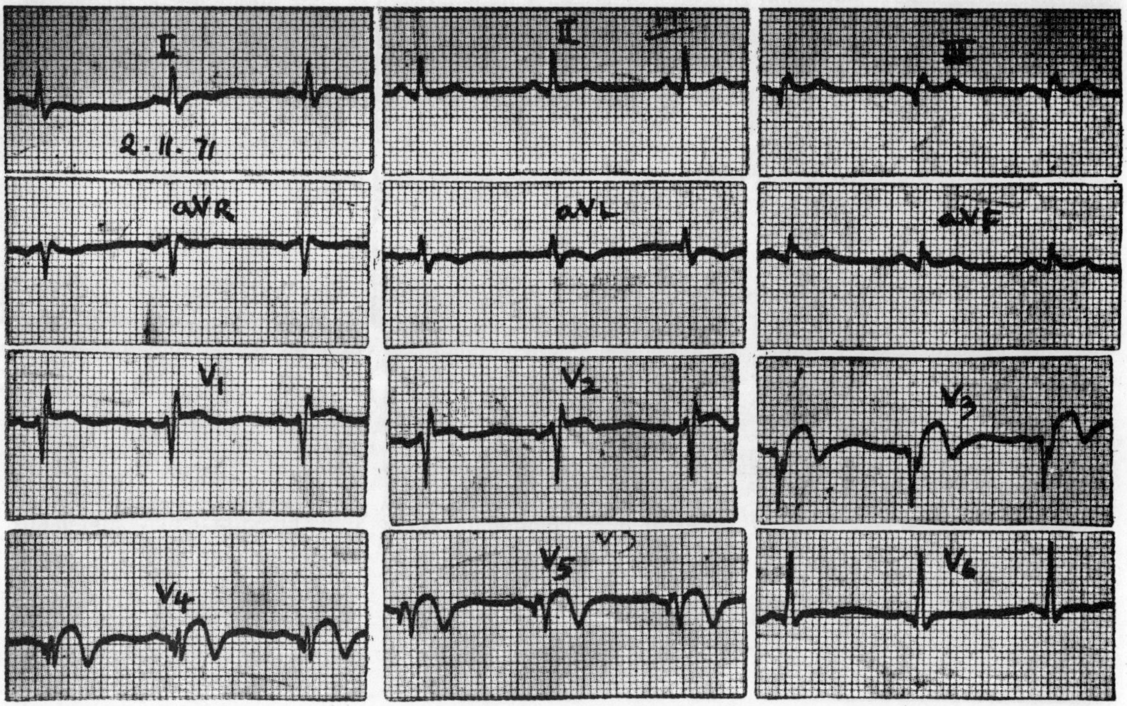

REVIEW TRACING 23.*

* For interpretation *vide* page 155

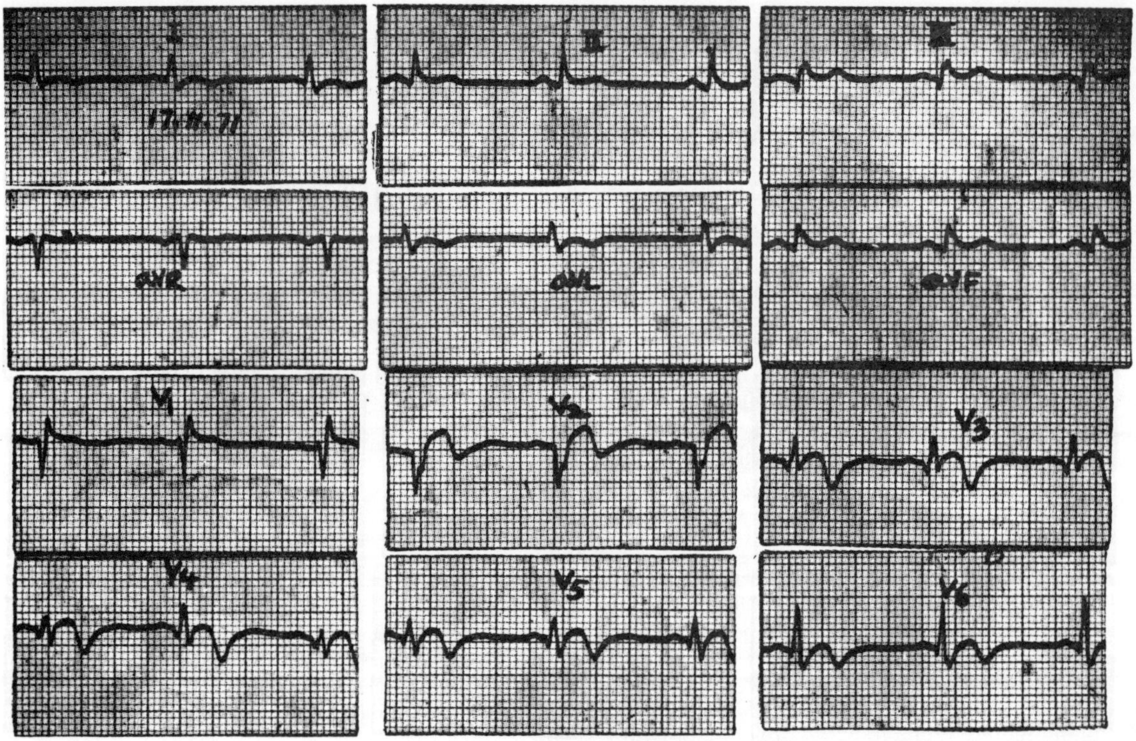

REVIEW TRACING 24.*

* For interpretation vide page 155

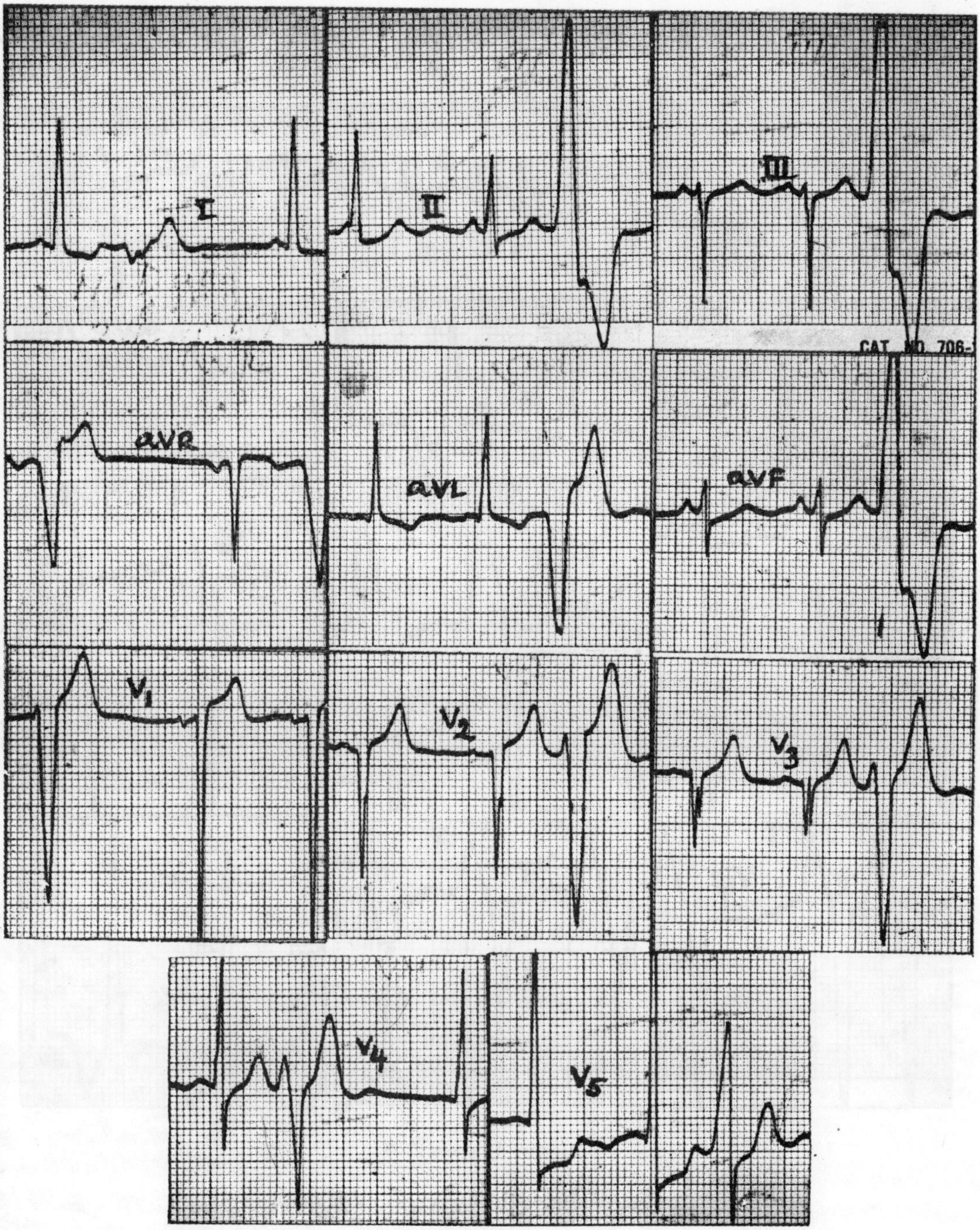

REVIEW TRACING 25.*

* For interpretation *vide* page 155

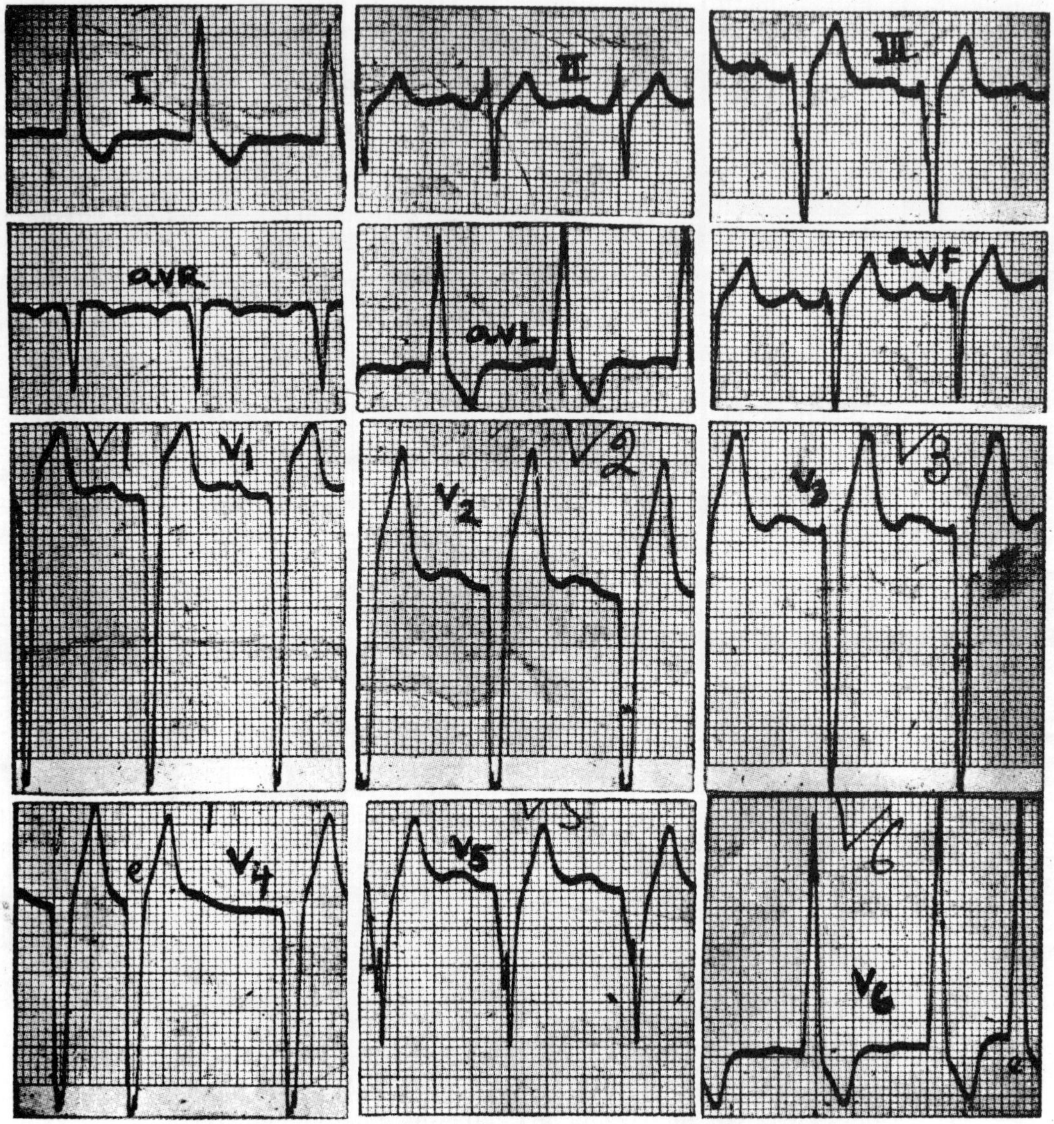

REVIEW TRACING 26.*

* For interpretation *vide* page 155

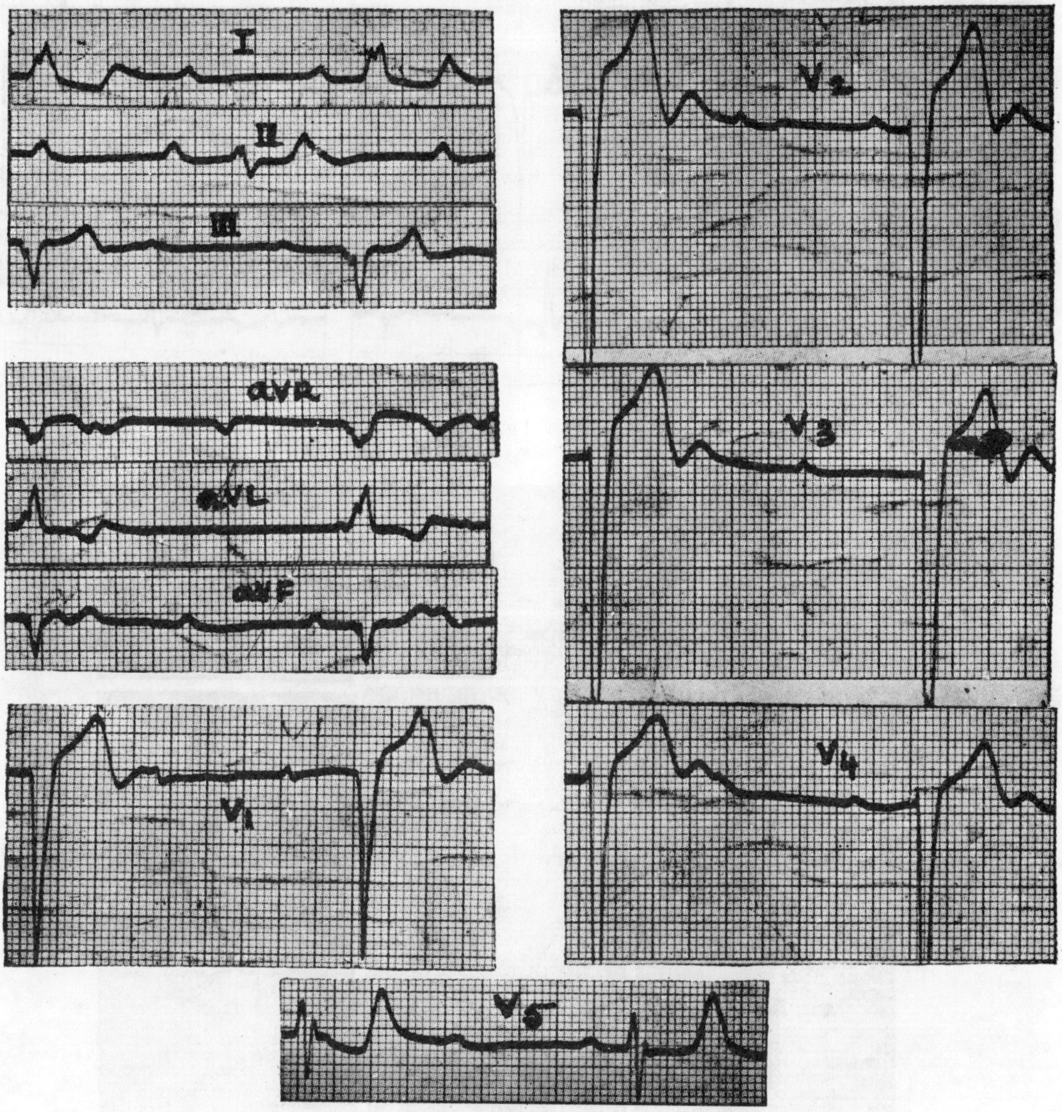

REVIEW TRACING 27.*

* For interpretation *vide* page 155

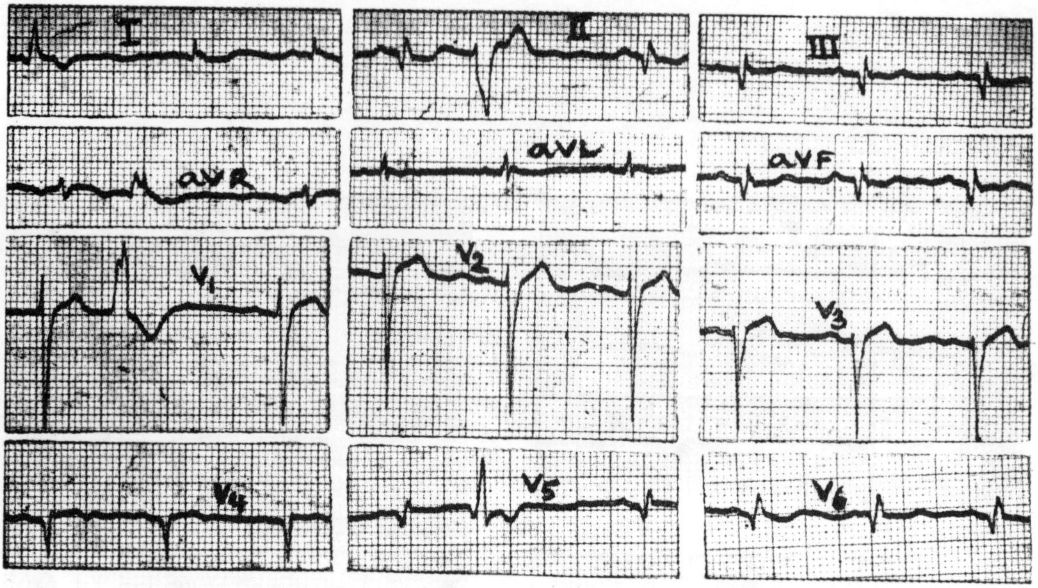

Review Tracing 28.*

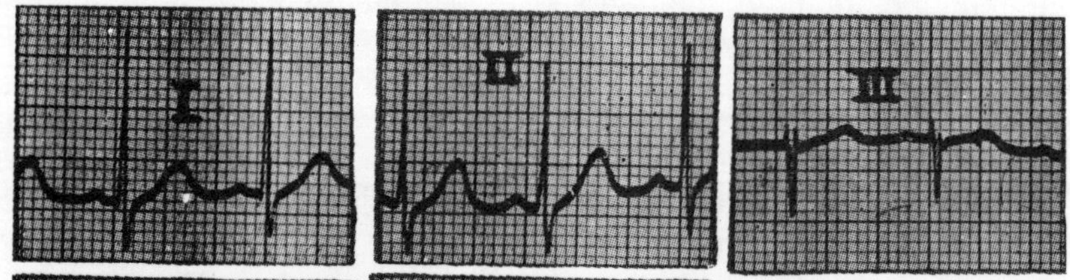

Review Tracing 29.**

* For interpretation *vide* page 155

** For interpretation *vide* page 156

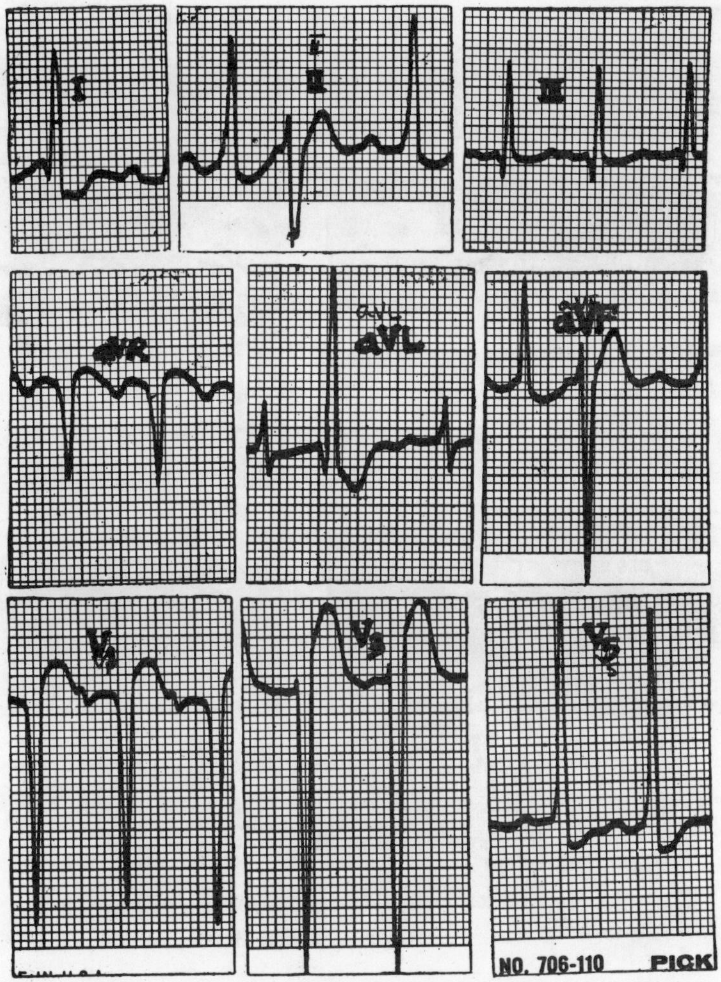

REVIEW TRACING 30.*

* For interpretation *vide* page 156

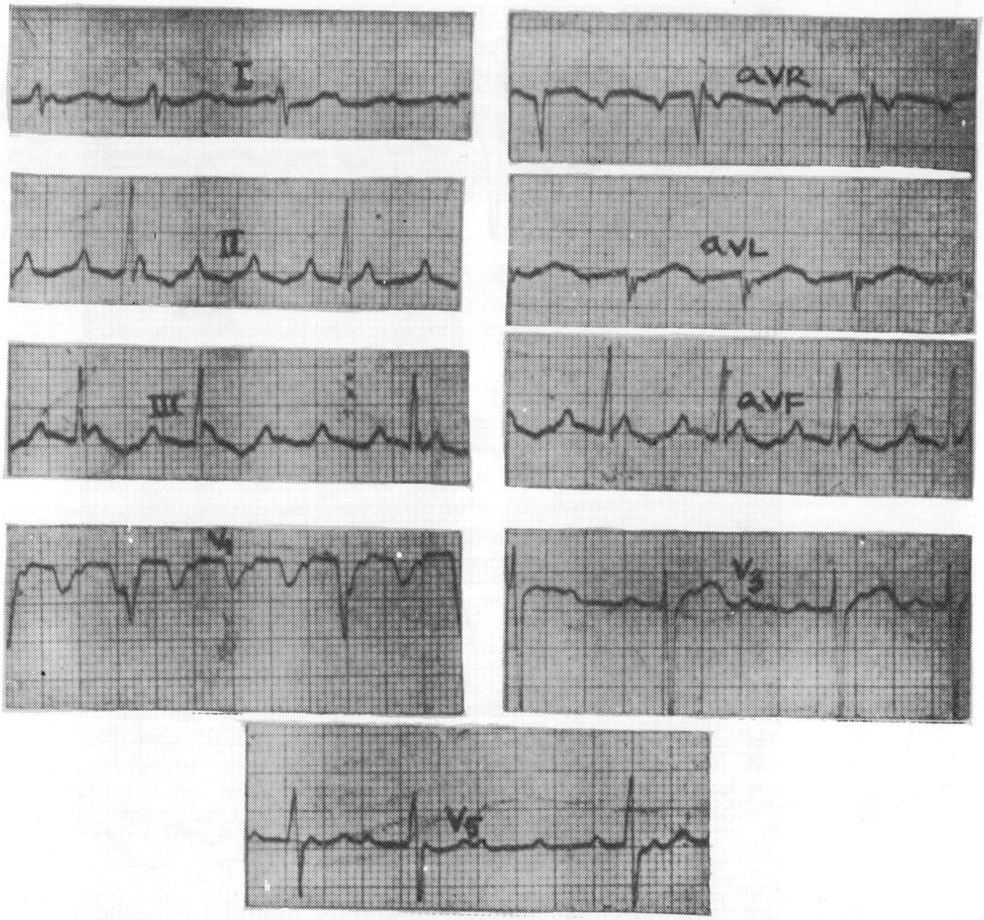

REVIEW TRACING 31.*

* For interpretation *vide* page 156

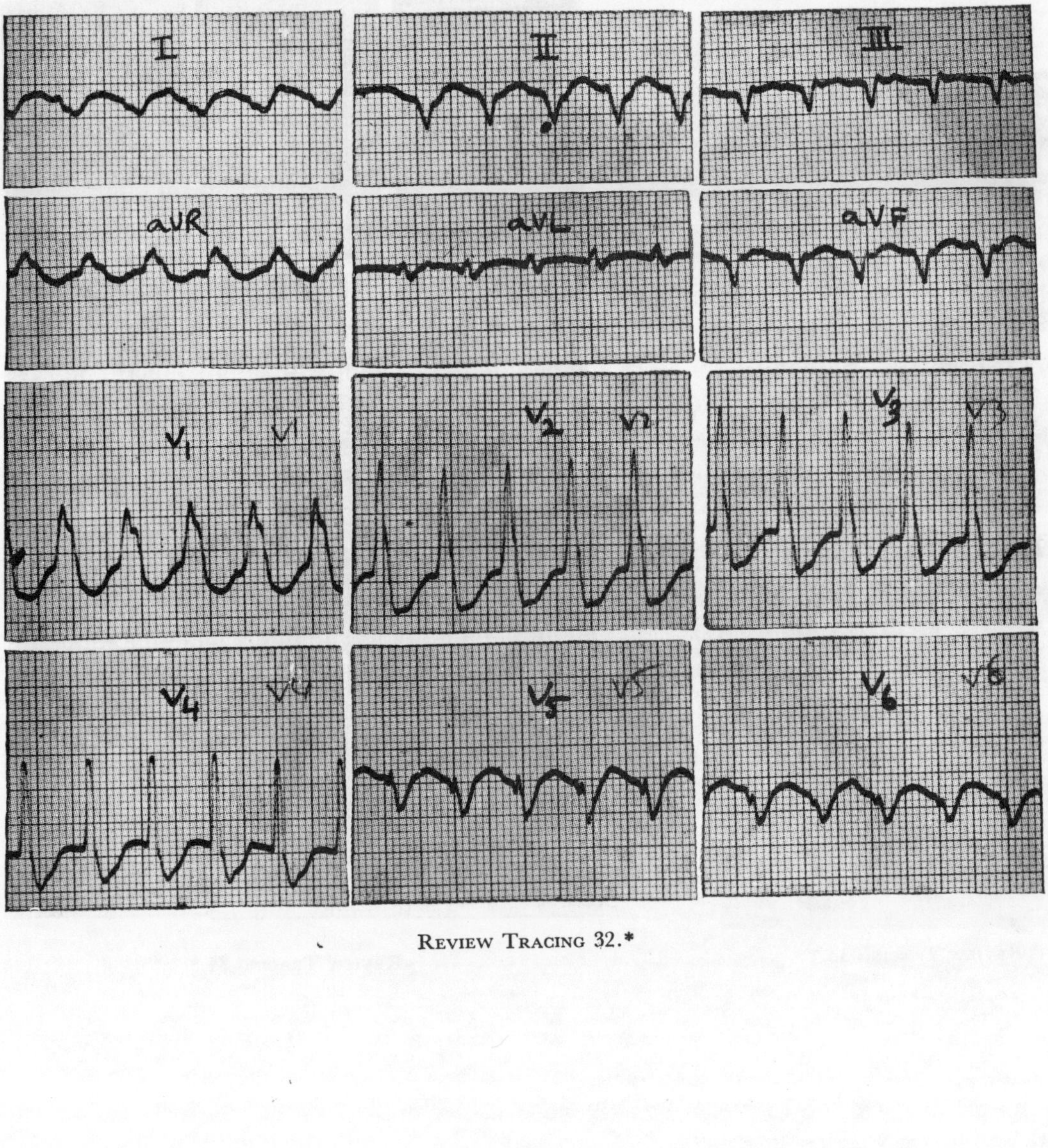

REVIEW TRACING 32.*

* For interpretation *vide* page 156

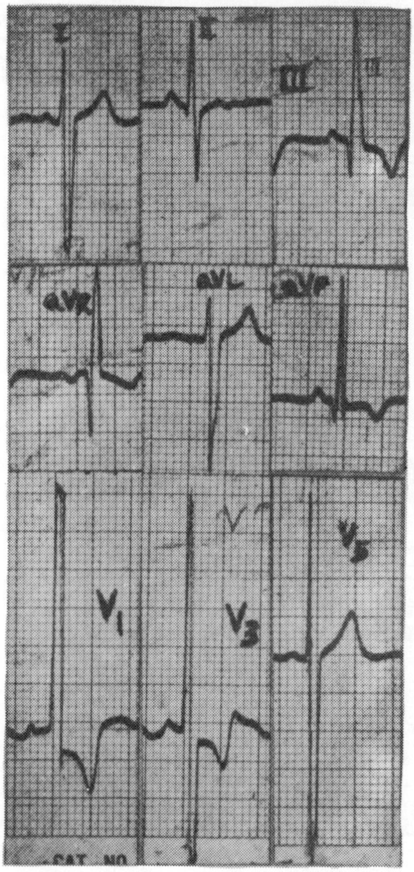

REVIEW TRACING 33.*

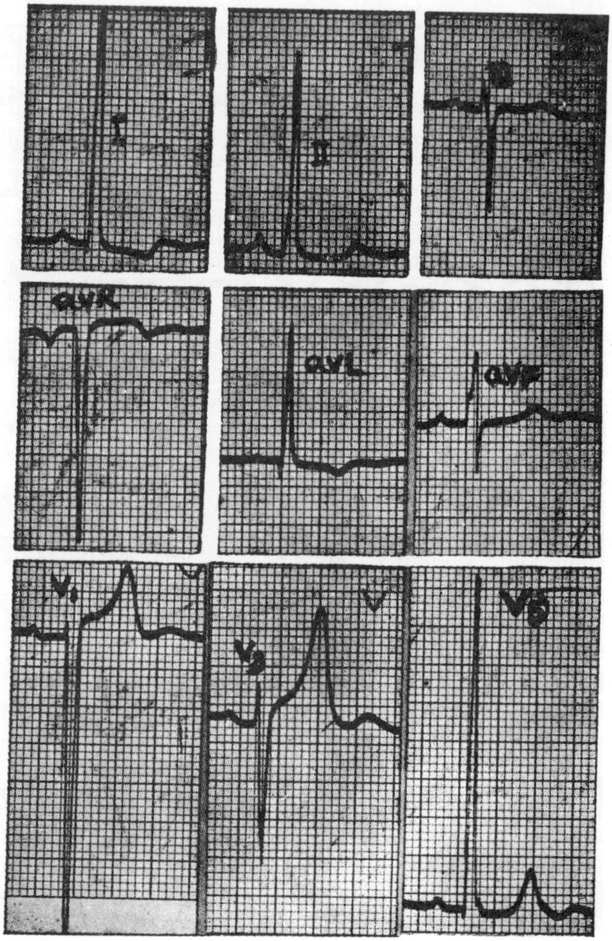

REVIEW TRACING 34.*

* For interpretation *vide* page 156

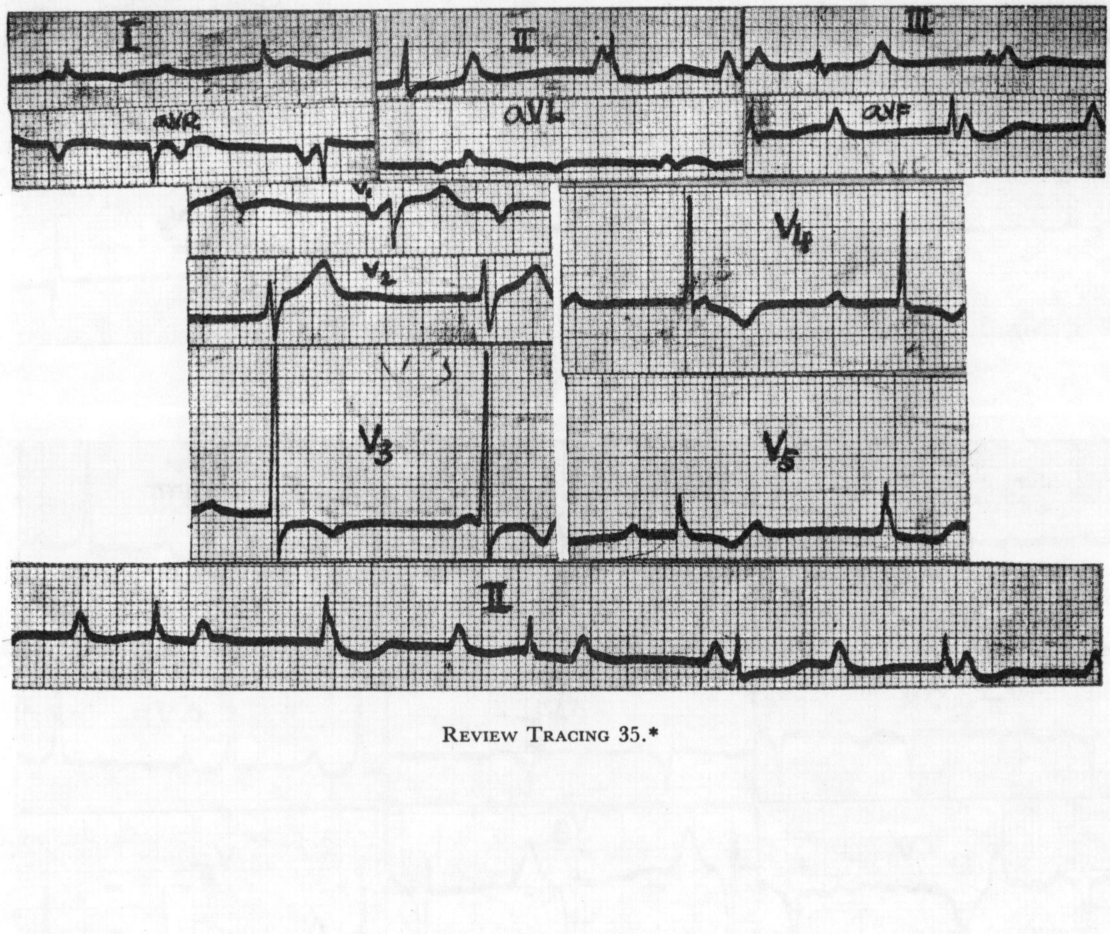

REVIEW TRACING 35.*

* For interpretation *vide* page 156

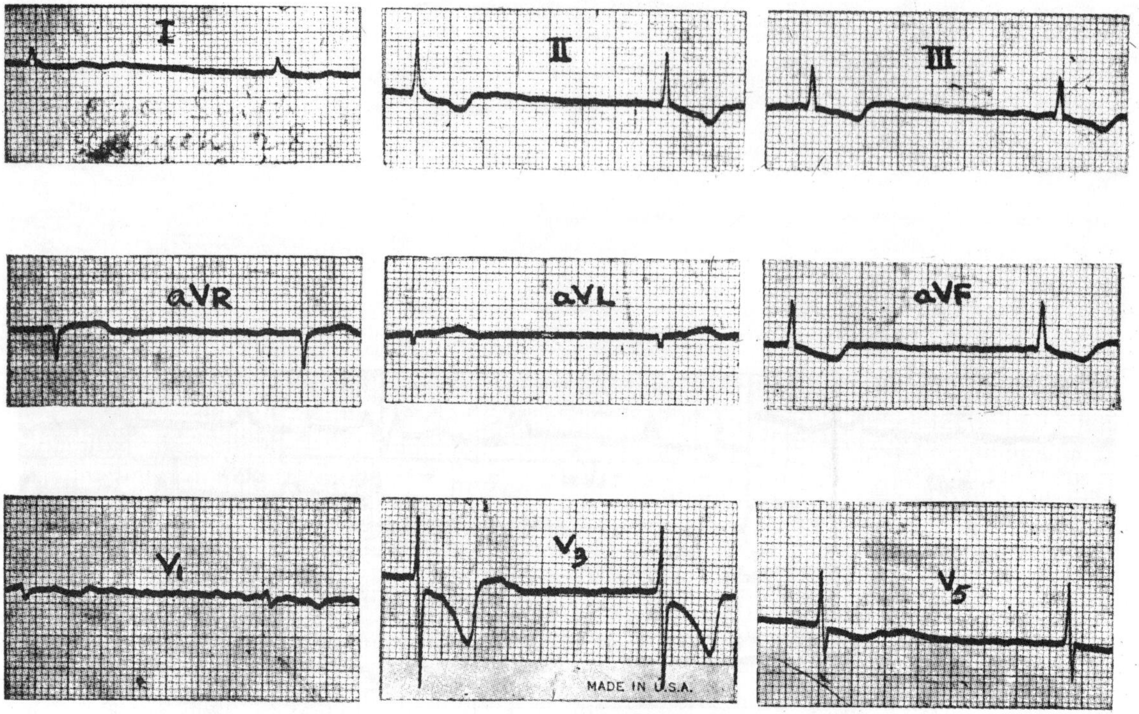

REVIEW TRACING 36.*

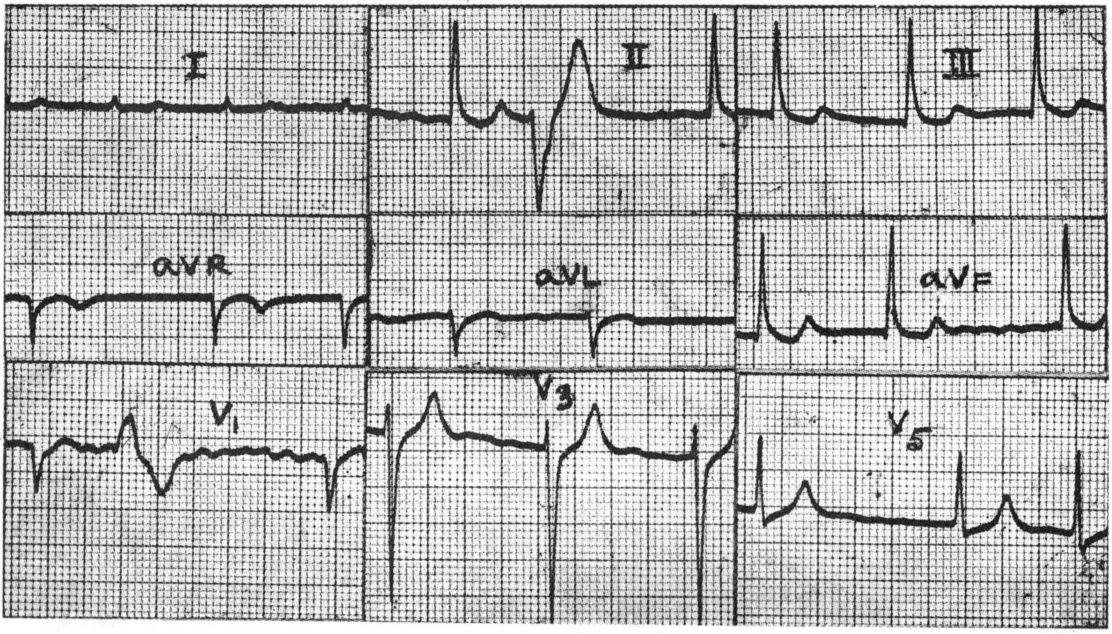

REVIEW TRACING 37.*

* For interpretation *vide* page 156

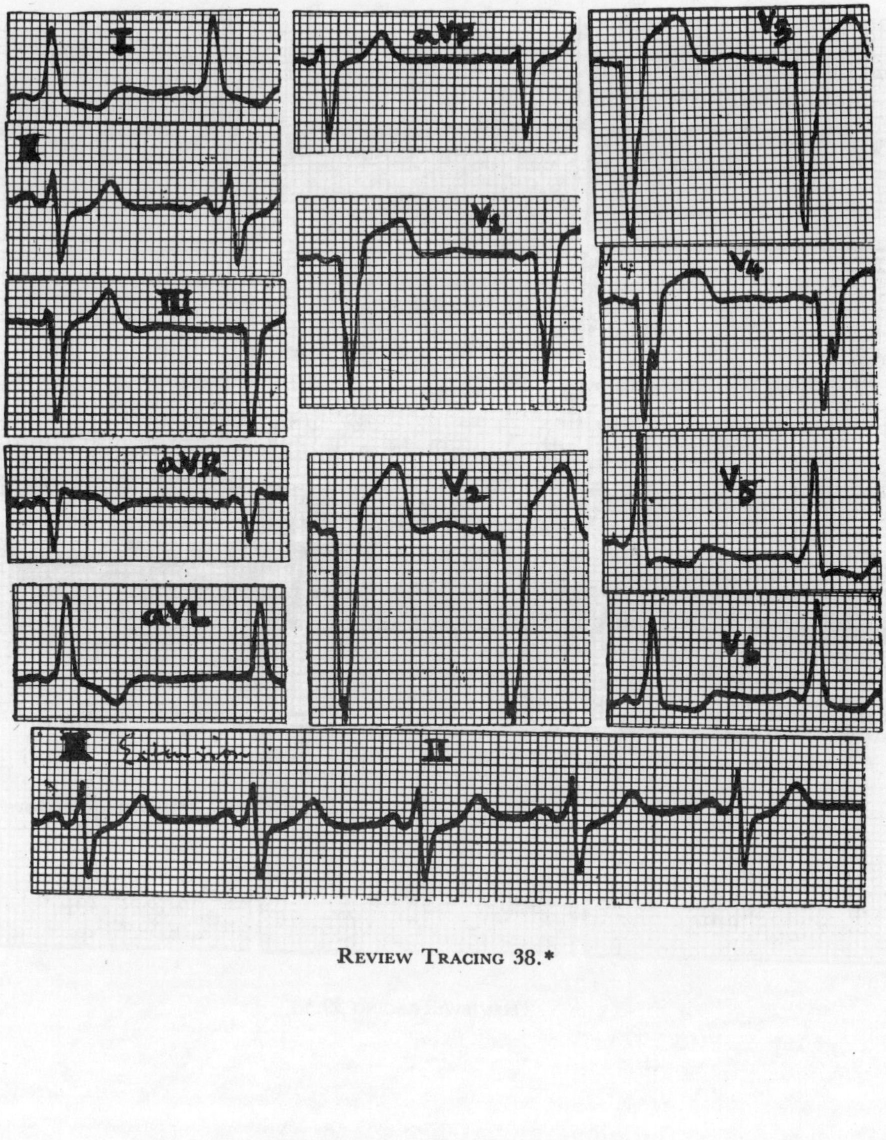

REVIEW TRACING 38.*

* For interpretation *vide* page 156

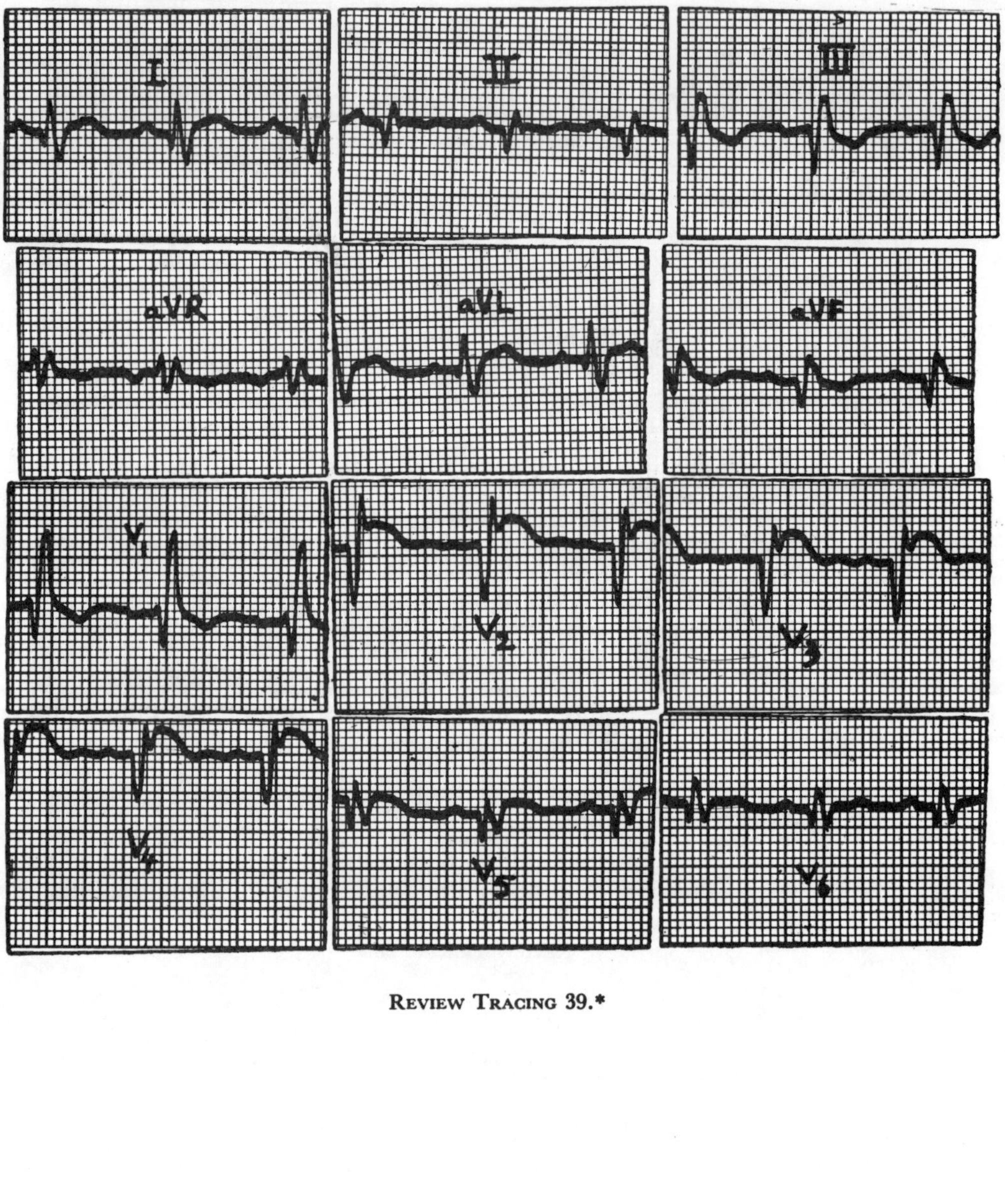

REVIEW TRACING 39.*

* For interpretation *vide* page 156

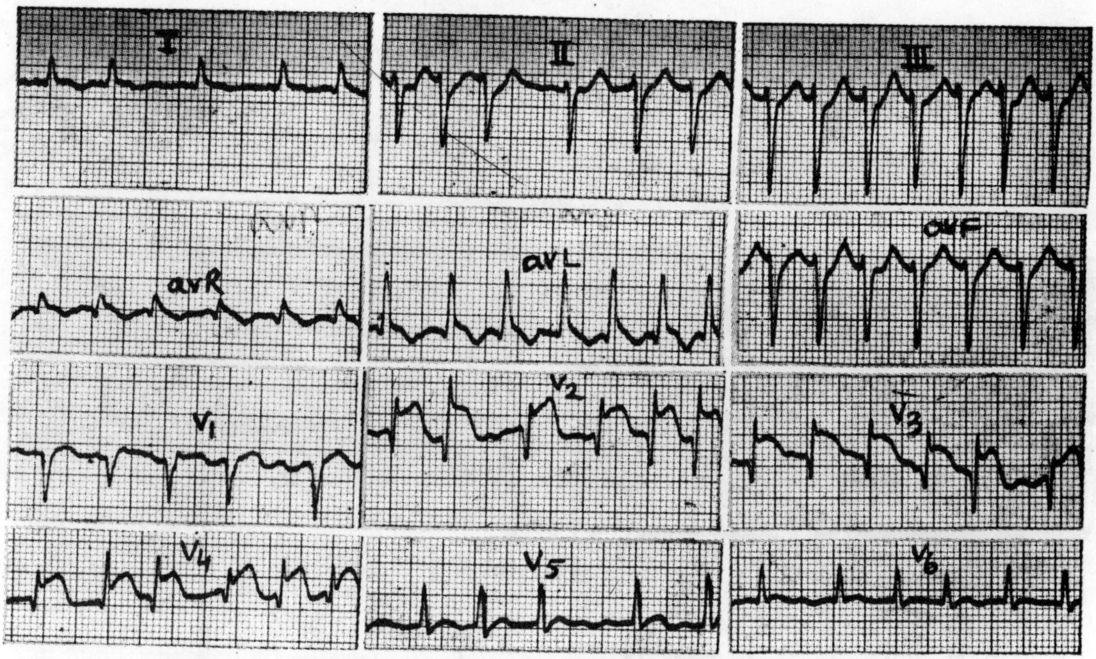

REVIEW TRACING 40.*

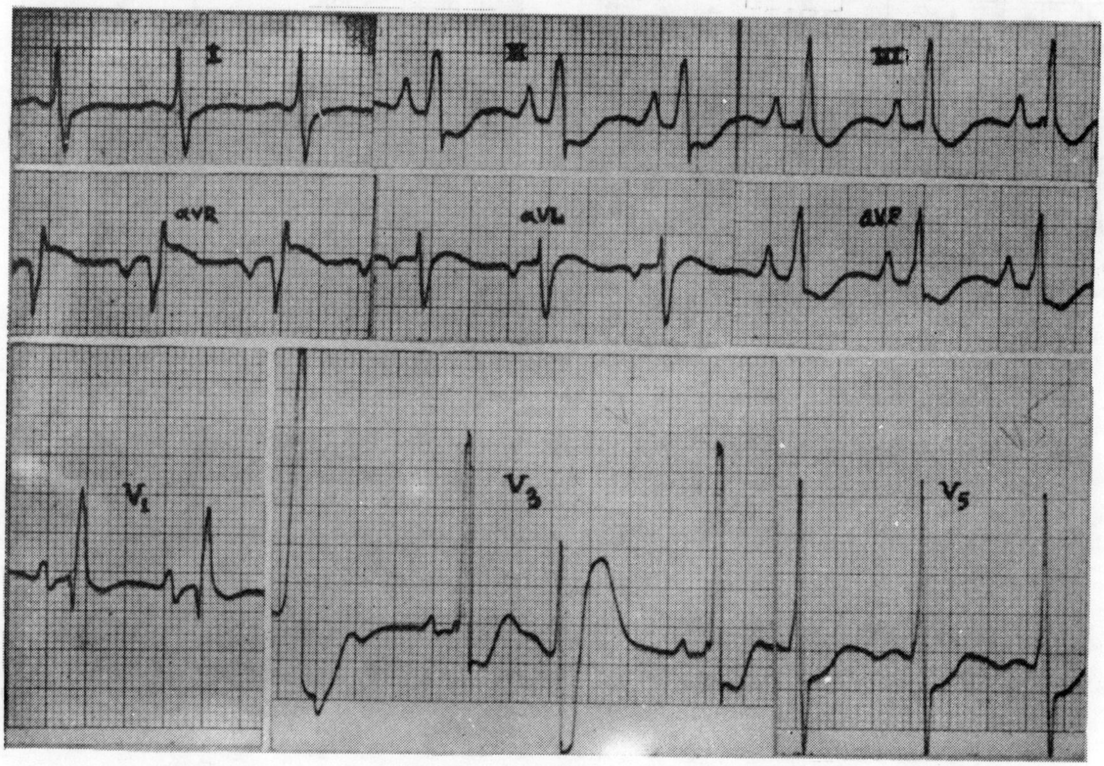

REVIEW TRACING 41.*

* For interpretation *vide* page 156

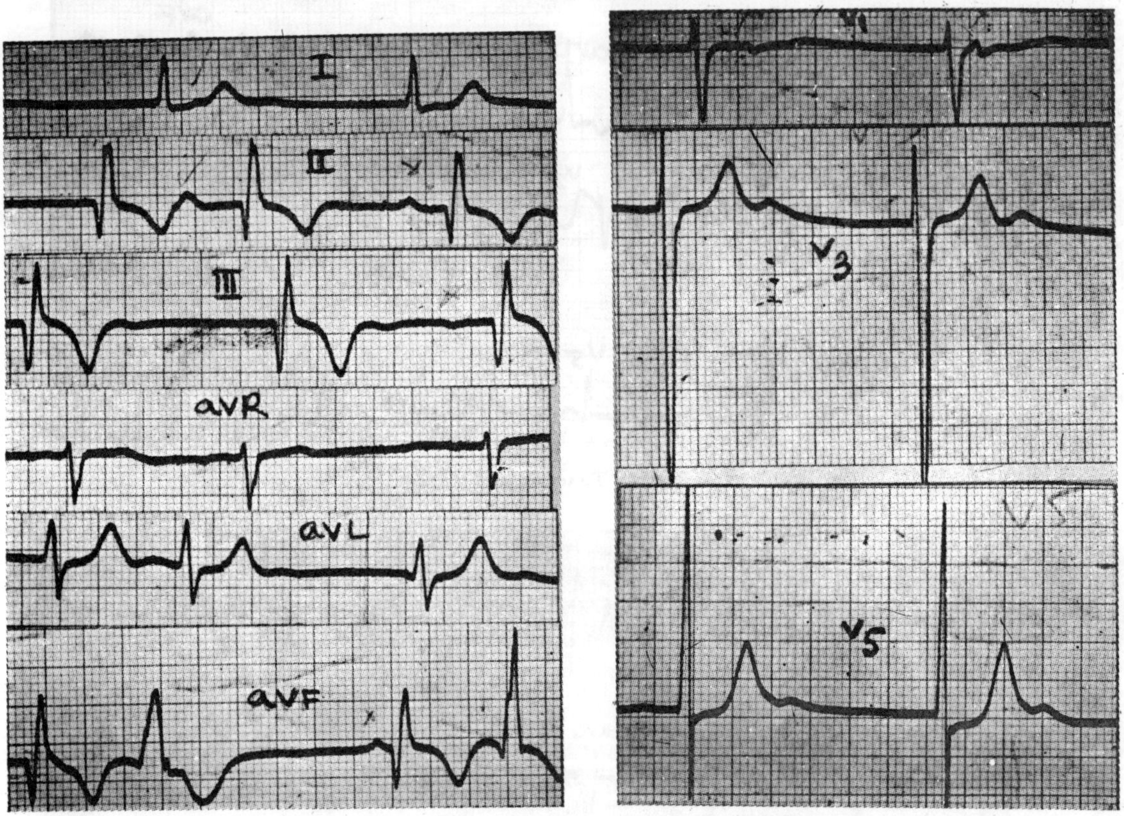

REVIEW TRACING 42.*

* For interpretation *vide* page 156

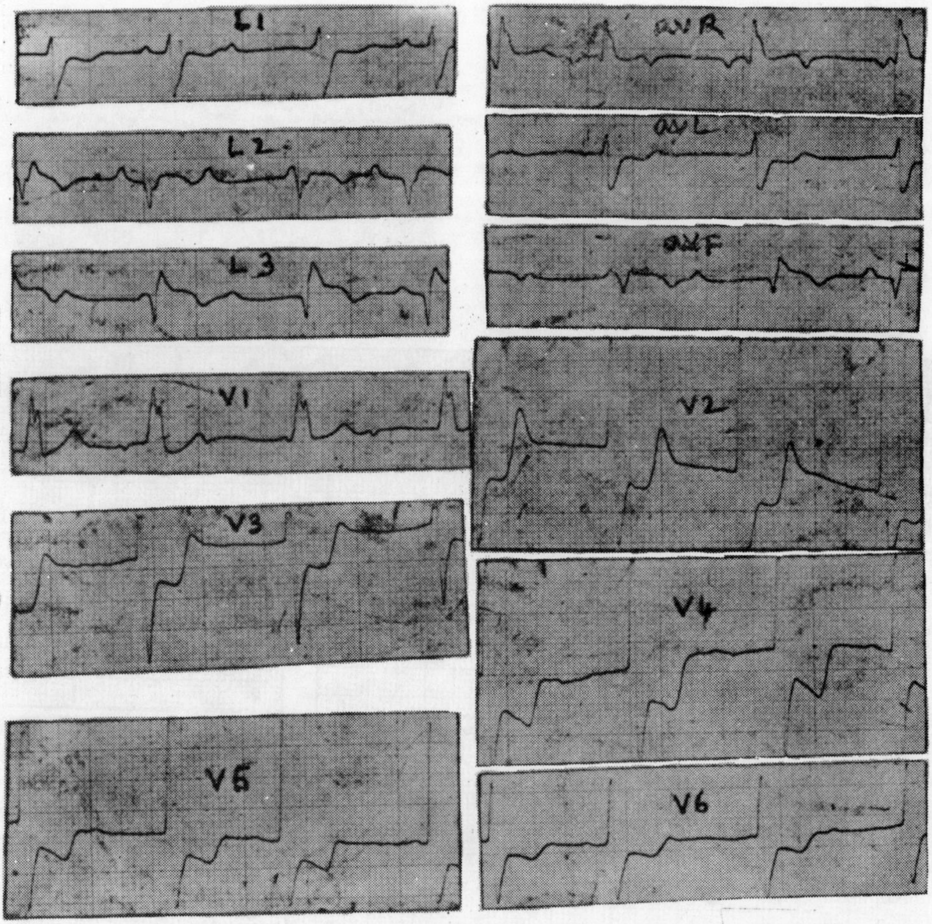

REVIEW TRACING 43.*

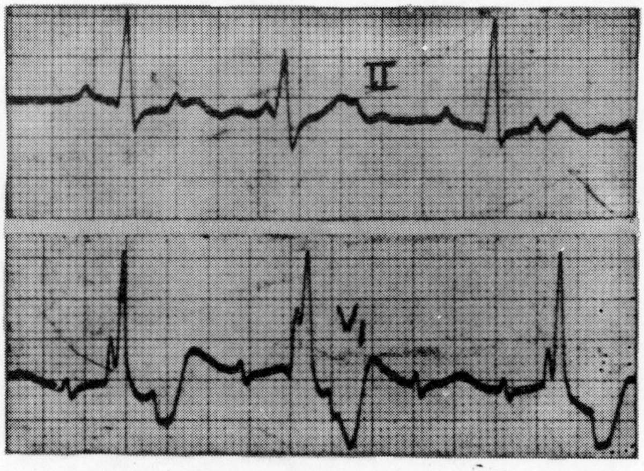

REVIEW TRACING 44.*

* For interpretations *vide* page 157

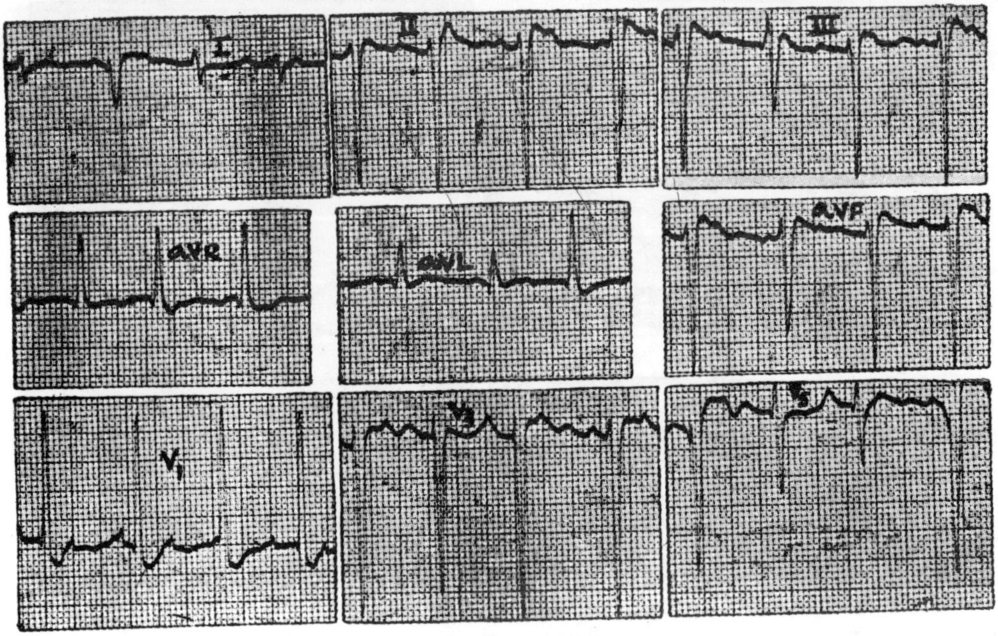

REVIEW TRACING 45.*

* For interpretation *vide* page 157

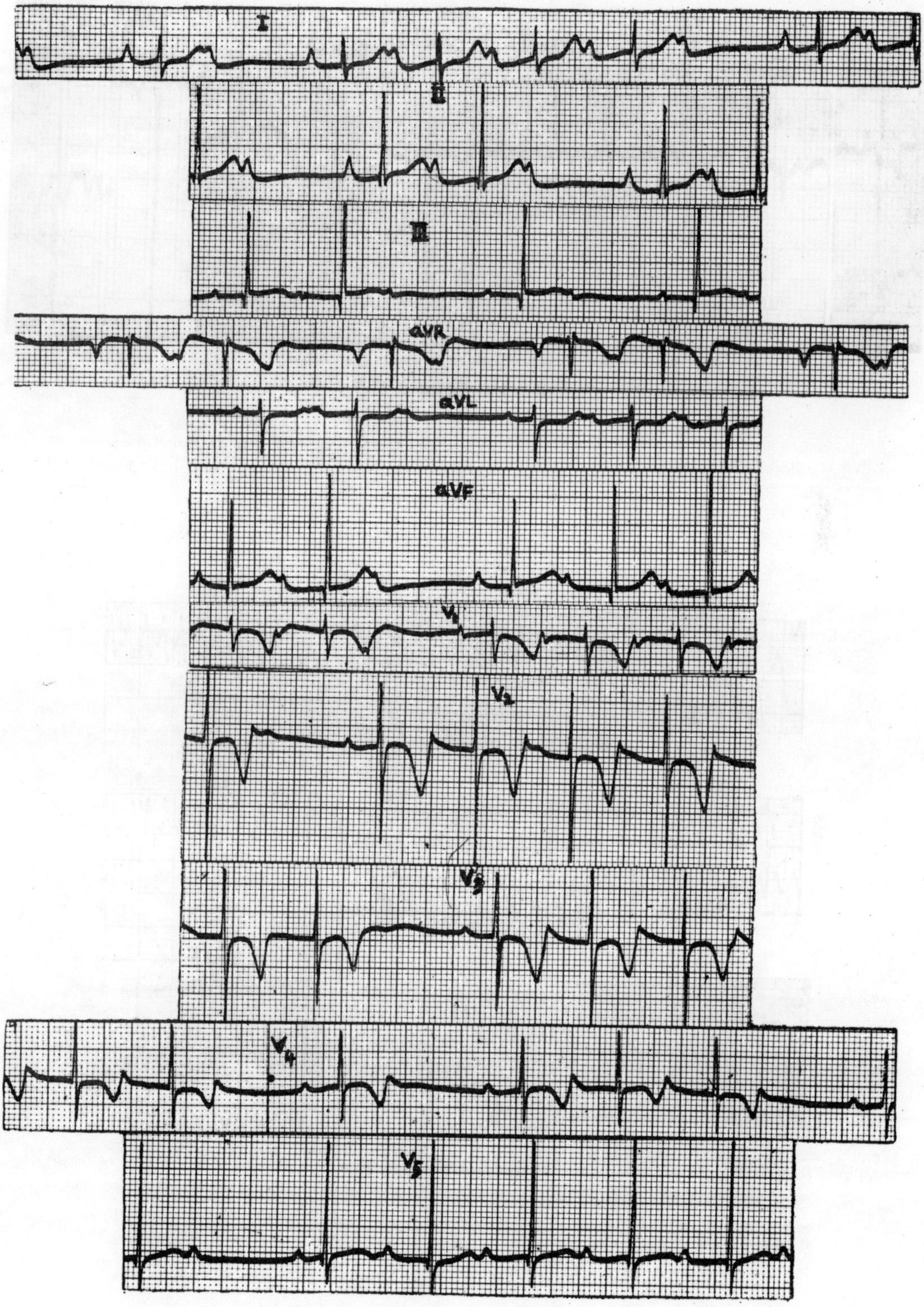

REVIEW TRACING 46.*

* For interpretation *vide* page 157

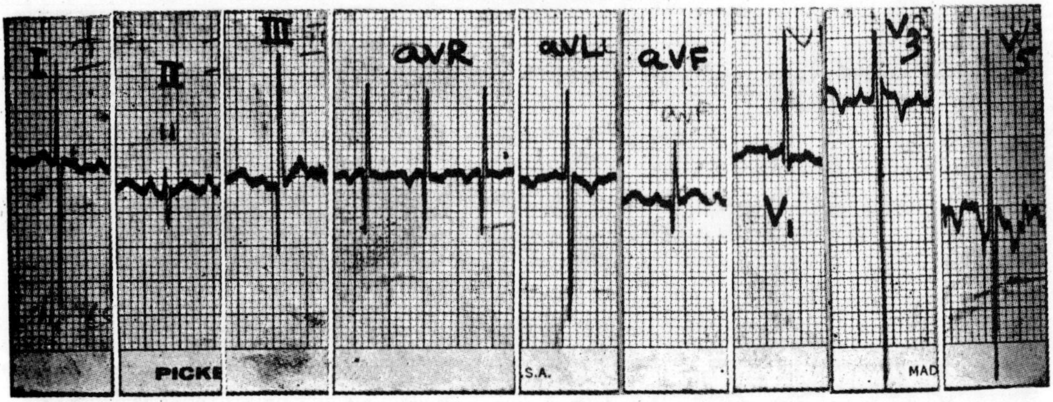

REVIEW TRACING 47.*

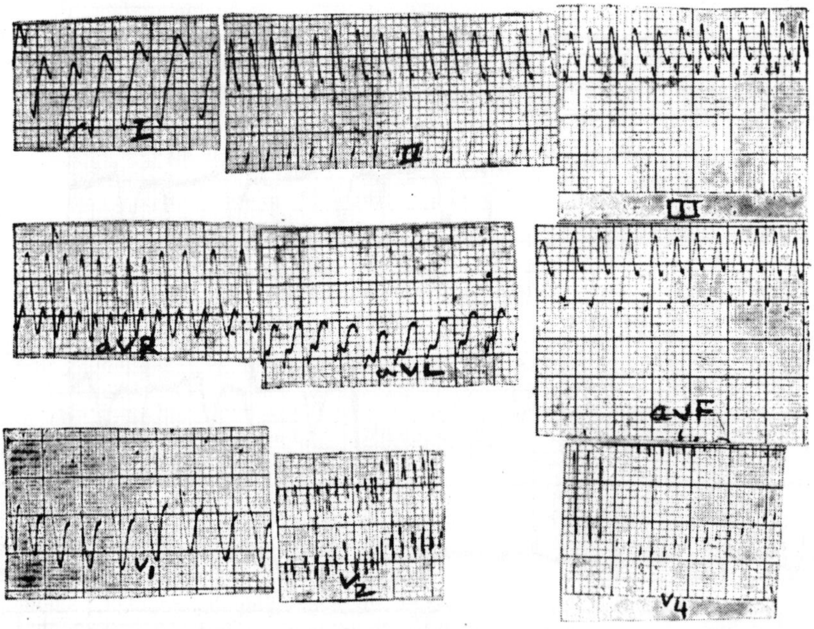

REVIEW TRACING 48.*

* For interpretations *vide* page 157

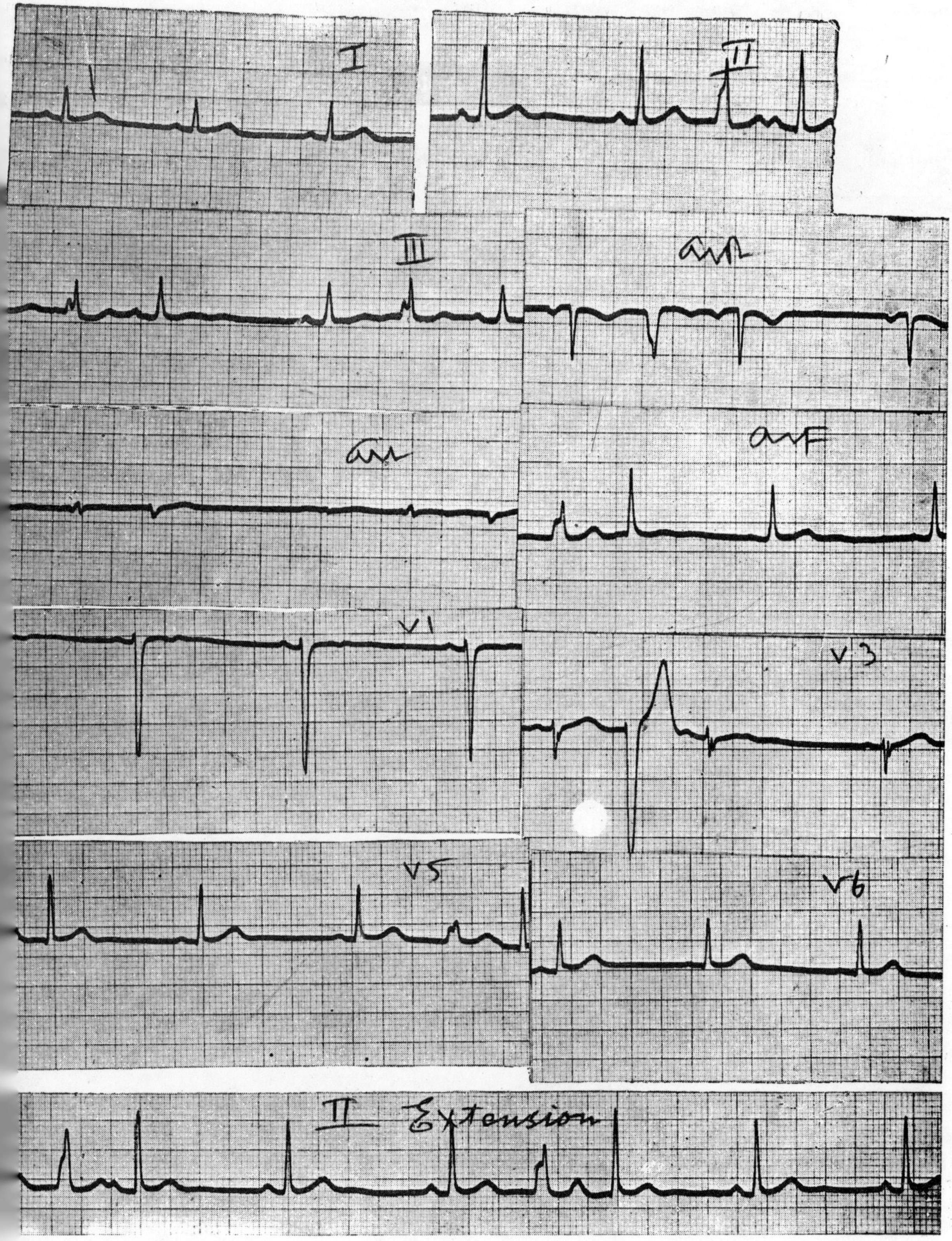

REVIEW TRACING 49.*

* For interpretation vide page 157

For Notes

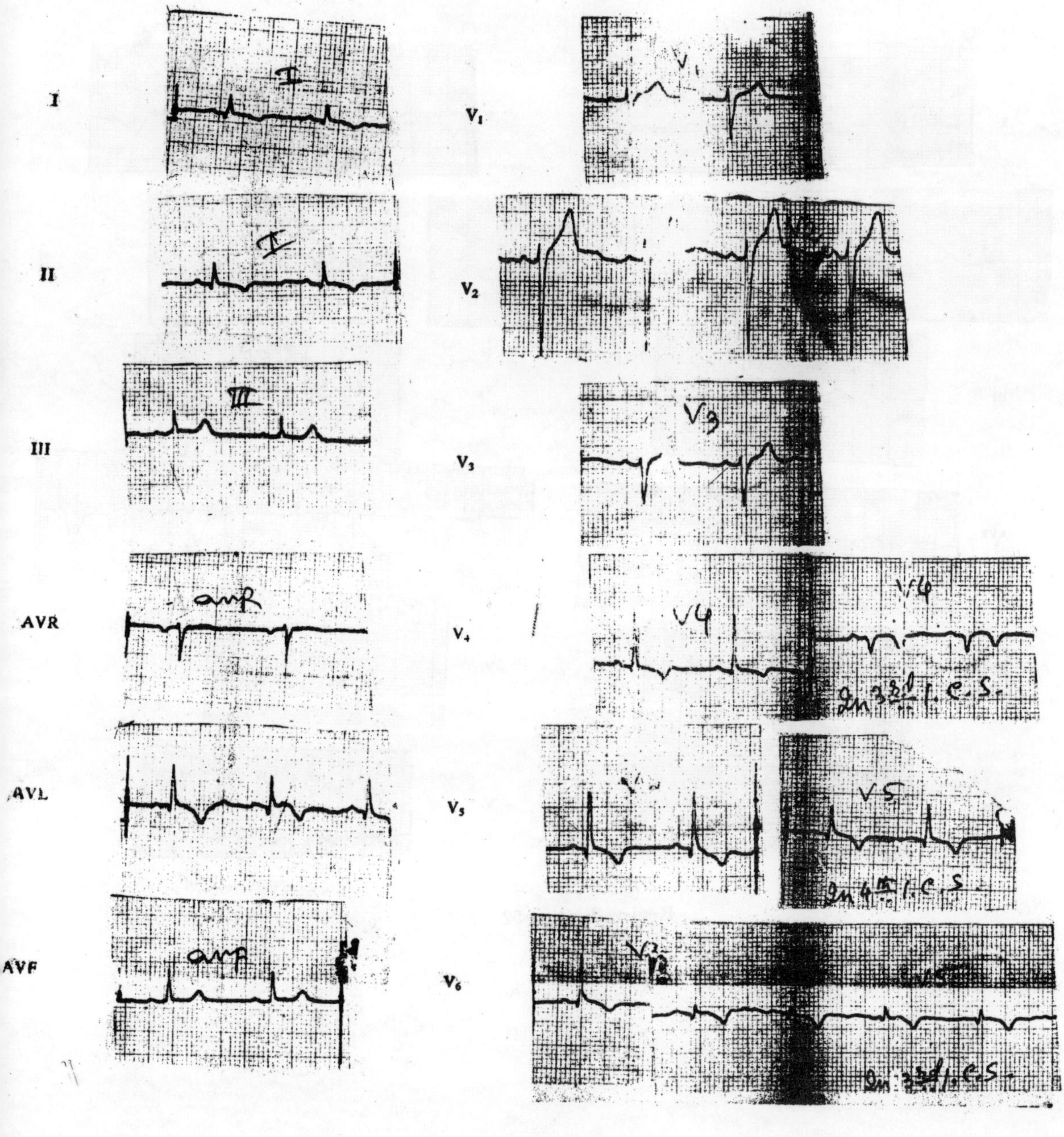

Review Tracing 51

* For interpretation *vide* Page 157

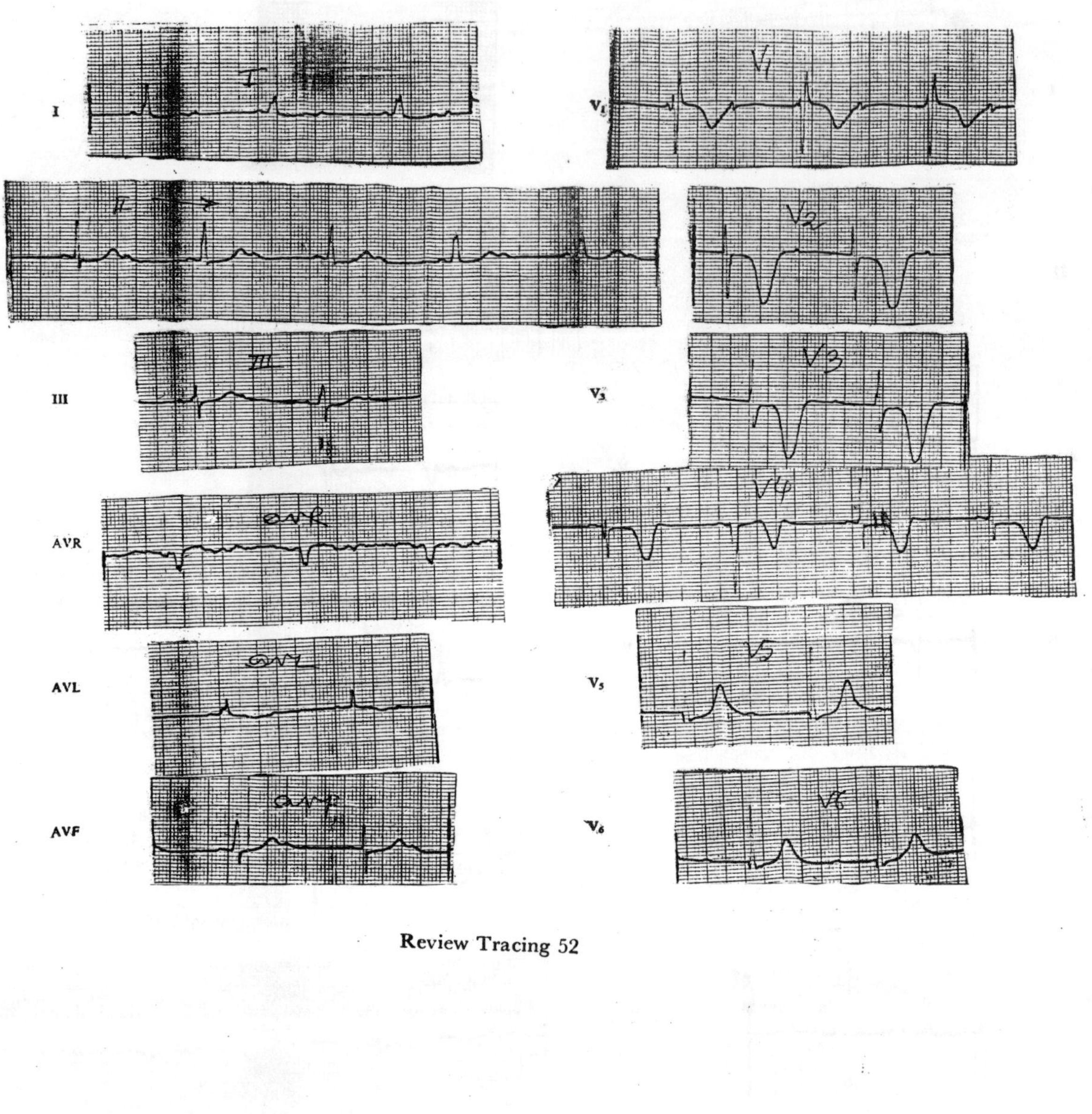

Review Tracing 52

* For interpretation *vide* Page 157

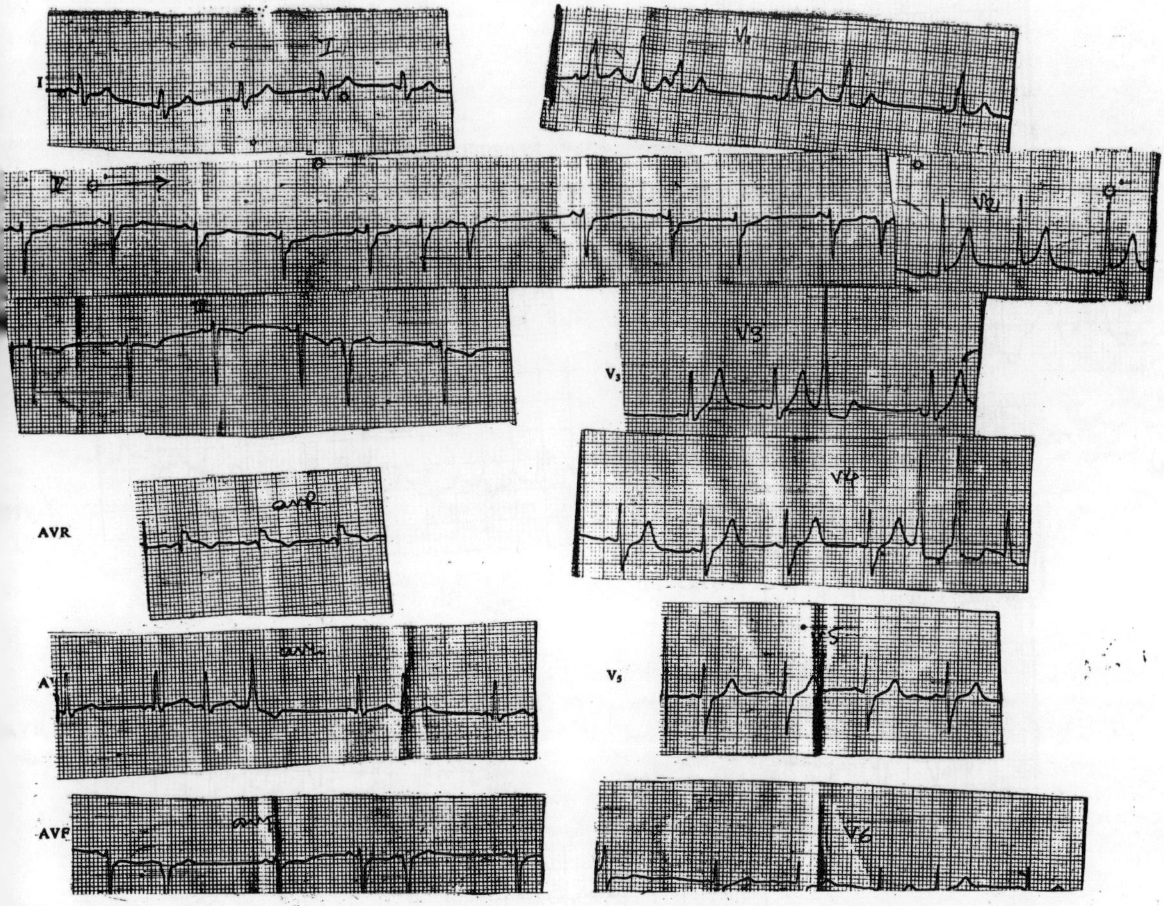

Review Tracing 53

• For interpretation *vide* Page 158

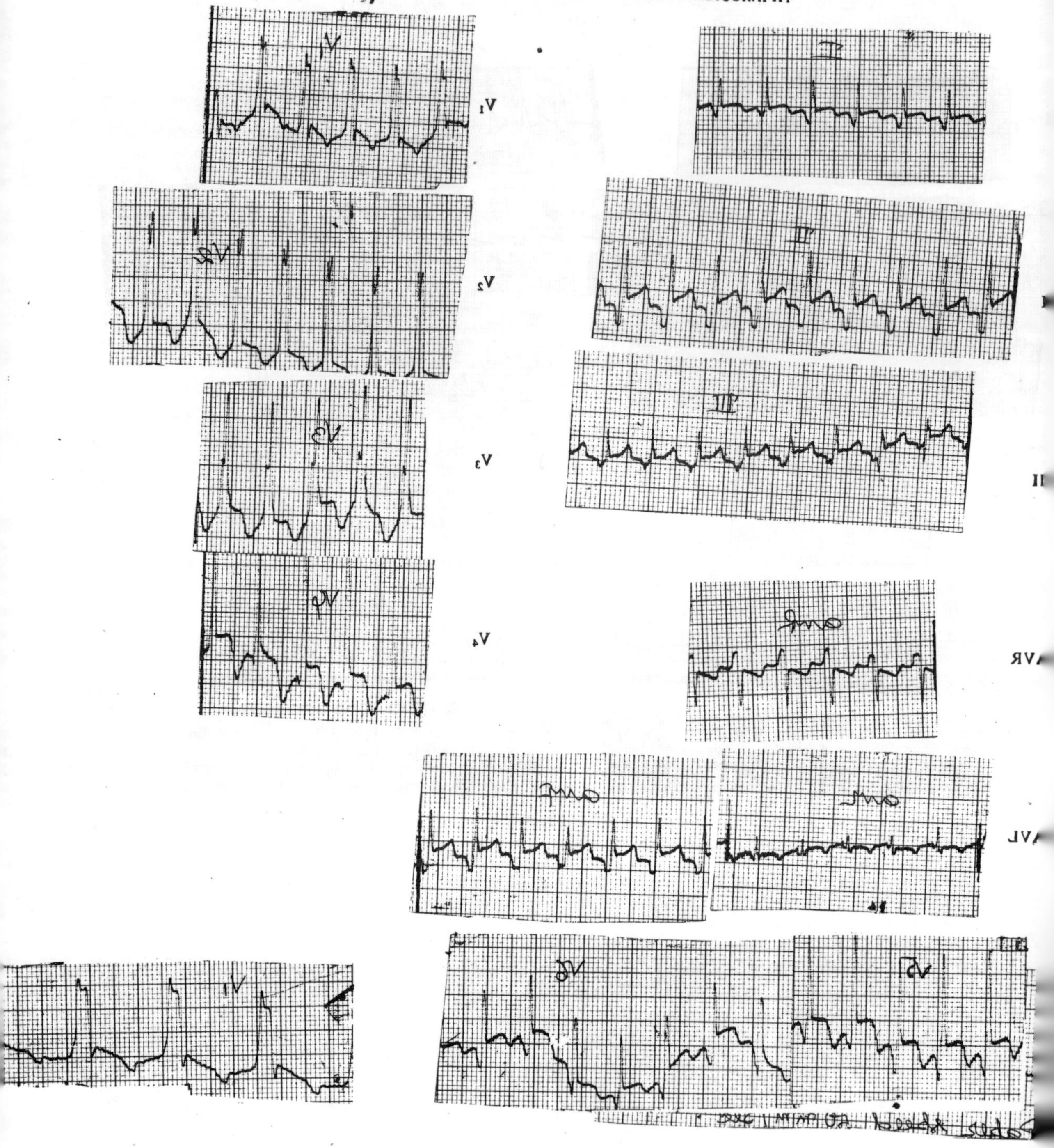

Review Tracing 54

* For interpretation *vide* Page 158

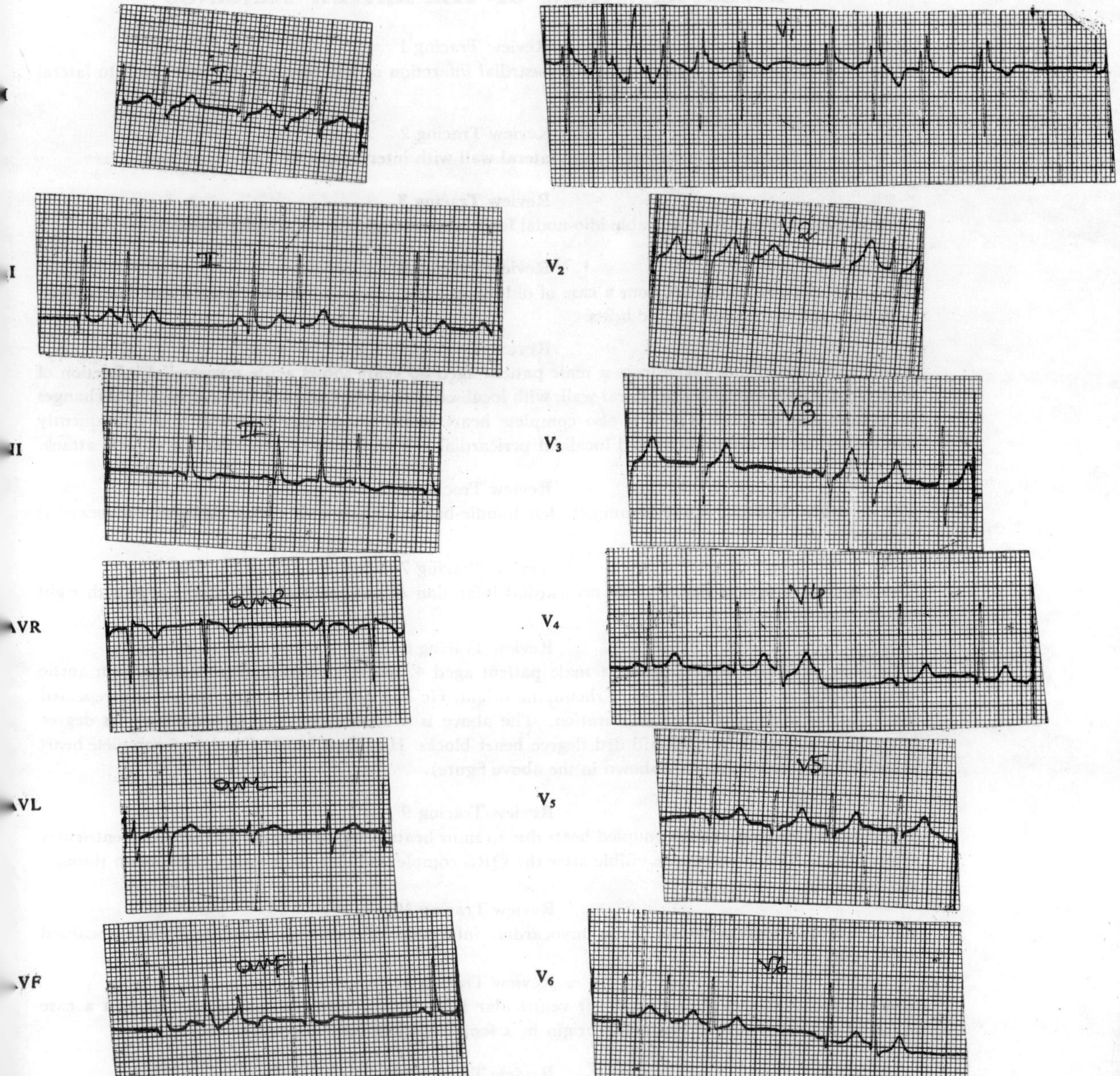

Review Tracing 55

* For interpretation *vide* Page 158

INTERPRETATIONS OF THE REVIEW TRACINGS

Review Tracing 1

This is a tracing from a case of recent myocardial infarction of anteroseptal wall spreading to lateral wall with right bundle-branch block.

Review Tracing 2

Myocardial infarction of anteroseptal and lateral wall with intermittent W.P.W. Syndrome.

Review Tracing 3

Complete heart block with unstable idio-nodal focus and intermittent ventricular standstill.

Review Tracing 4

This is an electrocardiogram from a case of old myocardial infarction of anteroseptal and lateral wall with frequent ventricular ectopic beats.

Review Tracing 5

This electrocardiogram taken from a male patient aged 58 years shows acute myocardial infarction of anteroseptal wall spreading to lateral wall, with localised pericarditis and ischaemic myocardial changes in postero-inferior wall. There is also complete heart block, ventricular standstill and subsequently cardiac standstill. The patient had localised pericardial rub and died 12 hrs. after the clinical attack.

Review Tracing 6

The electrocardiogram shows incomplete left bundle-branch block with diffuse ischaemic myocardial changes.

Review Tracing 7

The electrocardiogram shows acute myocardial infarction of anteroseptal and lateral wall with right bundle-branch block.

Review Tracing 8

This is an electrocardiogram from a male patient aged 42 years who had aortic stenosis with aortic incompetence and mitral stenosis of rheumatic origin. He had congestive cardiac failure and repeated Stock-Adams attacks of variable duration. The above is a continuous tracing and shows 1st degree heart block followed by 2nd and 3rd degree heart blocks. He subsequently developed complete heart block in the same tracing (not shown in the above figure).

Review Tracing 9

The electrocardiogram shows coupled beats due to sinus beats being alternately followed by ventricular ectopic beats. The P waves are visible after the QRS complexes due to retrograde conduction through the A-V node.

Review Tracing 10

The electrocardiogram shows acute myocardial infarction of postero-inferior wall with localised pericarditis.

Review Tracing 11

The electrocardiogram shows gross left ventricular hypertrophy with diastolic overloading in a case of mitral incompetence of rheumatic origin in a female patient aged 18 years.

Review Tracing 12

The electrocardiogram shows W.P.W. Syndrome in acquired heart disease; there is left ventricular hypertrophy and strain; the tracing has been taken from a male patient aged 60 years suffering from ischaemic heart disease.

Review Tracing 13

The electrocardiogram shows incomplete right bundle-branch block; there are frequent ventricular ectopic beats arising alternately from both the ventricles; there is also diffuse myocardial ischaemia. The patient aged 56 years complained of effort angina.

Review Tracing 14

The electrocardiogram shows acute transmural myocardial infarction of postero-inferior wall and acute subendocardial infarction of septal wall.

Review Tracing 15

The electrocardiogram shows old myocardial infarction of postero-inferior wall, with slow atrial fibrillation.

Review Tracing 16

The electrocardiogram shows myocardial infarction of some duration of septal wall, ischaemic changes in anterolateral wall with frequent ventricular ectopic beats.

Review Tracing 17

The electrocardiogram shows subendocardial infarction of septal wall spreading to lateral wall with right bundle-branch block and left ventricular hypertrophy. There is also an evidence of *cardiac ancurysm* in postero-inferior wall. The patient had acute myocardial infarction in the postero-inferior wall 8 months ago when there was no right bundle-branch block.

Review Tracing 18

The electrocardiogram shows subacute myocardial infarction of anteroseptal and lateral wall spreading to postero-inferior wall. The tracing was taken 12 hours after the onset of precordial pain. There was no past history of precordial pain.

Review Tracing 19

The electrocardiogram shows recent myocardial infarction of anteroseptal and lateral wall. There is also old myocardial infarction of postero-inferior wall.

Review Tracing 20

The electrocardiogram shows low voltage complexes due to extensive myocardial disease. There is old myocardial infarction of anteroseptal and lateral wall and myocardial ischaemia in postero-inferior wall. There is also a nodal ectopic beat with delayed conduction in lead V_5.

Review Tracing 21

The electrocardiogram shows subepicardial infarction of septal wall spreading to lateral wall.

Review Tracing 22

The electrocardiogram shows recent myocardial infarction of septal and lateral wall with spread to anterior wall which was taken 2 weeks after the previous tracing (Review Tracing 21). There is also an evidence of right bundle-branch block.

Review Tracing 23

This electrocardiogram was taken 2 weeks after the previous tracing (Review Tracing 22) and shows recent myocardial infarction of septal and lateral wall with right bundle-branch block. There are also changes in QRS complexes suggestive of transmural myocardial infarction.

Review Tracing 24

This electrocardiogram was taken 2 weeks after the previous Tracing 23 (i.e. 42 days after the 1st tracing, i.e., Review Tracing 21) and shows a pattern of myocardial infarction of some duration of anteroseptal and lateral wall with persistence of right bundle-branch block.

Review Tracing 25

The electrocardiogram shows one ventricular ectopic beat after two sinus beats giving rise to pulsus trigeminus. There is also subendocardial infarction of lateral wall and gross left ventricular hypertrophy.

Review Tracing 26

The electrocardiogram shows complete left bundle-branch block with old myocardial infarction of anteroseptal and lateral wall. There is also considerably widened P wave indicating intra-atrial block. In lead V_4 there is a nodal ectopic beat and in lead V_5 there is aberrant ventricular conduction.

Review Tracing 27

The electrocardiogram shows complete heart block with established idio-ventricular rhythm and left ventricular hypertrophy.

Review Tracing 28

The electrocardiogram shows old myocardial infarction of postero-inferior, anteroseptal and lateral wall with frequent ventricular ectopic beats.

Review Tracing 29

This electrocardiogram was taken from a little girl aged 8 years who had atrial septal defect (ostium primum type). There is incomplete right bundle-branch block, right ventricular strain (overloading), left axis deviation and left ventricular hypertrophy.

Review Tracing 30

The electrocardiogram shows acute myocardial infarction of septal wall, subendocardial infarction in anterolateral wall and myocardial ischaemia in postero-inferior wall, frequent atrial ectopic beats and left ventricular hypertrophy.

Review Tracing 31

The tracing shows Atrial Flutter with varying grades of heart block giving rise to an irregular rhythm. The atrial rate is relatively slow (atrial rate 200 per minute) with intermittent intra-atrial block.

Review Tracing 32

The electrocardiogram shows paroxysmal supraventricular tachycardia with intermittent bundle-branch block with old myocardial infarction of postero-inferior and anterolateral wall.

Review Tracing 33

The electrocardiogram shows gross right ventricular hypertrophy and strain (overloading) in a case of severe valvular pulmonary stenosis.

Review Tracing 34

The electrocardiogram shows gross left ventricular hypertrophy and strain (overloading) in a case of hypertension.

Review Tracing 35

The electrocardiogram shows complete heart block with idio-nodal rhythm, right atrial enlargement, diffuse ischaemic myocardial changes and ectopic QRS complexes in leads III, aVR, and II (bottom strip).

Review Tracing 36

This is an electrocardiogram showing diffuse ischaemic myocardial changes, complete heart block with idio-nodal rhythm and atrial fibrillation.

Review Tracing 37

The electrocardiogram shows atrial fibrillation with irregular ventricular rhythm and ventricular ectopic beats.

Review Tracing 38

The electrocardiogram shows acute myocardial infarction of septal wall with myocardial ischaemia in the lateral wall with left atrial enlargement and W.P.W. Syndrome.

Review Tracing 39

This is an electrocardiogram from a male patient aged 58 years who had a history of acute chest pain 2 years ago. The patient developed acute pain over the praecordium again after 2 years and the above electrocardiogram was taken 12 hours after the onset of chest pain. The electrocardiogram shows acute myocardial infarction of anteroseptal and lateral wall with right bundle-branch block and also an evidence of old myocardial infarction of postero-inferior wall.

Review Tracing 40

The electrocardiogram shows acute myocardial infarction in the septal wall with atrial fibrillation.

Review Tracing 41

This is a tracing from a patient aged 68 years who came with congestive cardiac failure. The tracing shows subendocardial infarction of septal and lateral wall and myocardial ischaemia in the postero-inferior wall. There is right bundle-branch block, right atrial enlargement and ventricular ectopic beats.

Review Tracing 42

The electrocardiogram shows myocardial infarction of some duration in the postero-inferior wall. There is nodal rhythm with increasingly delayed retrograde conduction giving rise to occasional reciporcal rhythm. In lead aVF there are two ventricular ectopic beats arising from two different foci. The two upright P waves (one in lead II and the other in lead aVF) are due to excitations from S-A node and may have captured the ventricles. There is also left ventricular hypertrophy.

Review Tracing 43

Myocardial infarction postero-inferior wall, sinus rhythm interrupted by blocked atrial ectopic beat followed by nodal escape, complete right bundle branch block.

Review Tracing 44

Complete heart block with unstable idioventricular focus.

Review Tracing 45

The E.C.G. shows a phenomenon of interference-dissociation. There is an accelerated idio-nodal rhythm with capture beats (interference beats) with aberrant conduction at times (top strips 2nd, 7th and 12th, middle strips 3rd, 5th and 10th, bottom strips 4th, 8th, 9th and 12th are interference beats), there is also right bundle branch block.

Review Tracing 46

Partial A–V heart block showing mostly Wenckebach's phenomena with irregularly dropped ventricular complexes; there is also ischaemic myocardial changes in the septal wall.

Review Tracing 47

The tracing shows supraventricular tachycardia, left ventricular hypertrophy, right ventricular dominance and strain, slow myocardial infarction postero-inferior wall, ischaemic myocardial changes anterolateral wall.

Review Tracing 48

The patient aged 50 years, male, had an acute myocardial infarction; he developed an arrhythmia which was an wonderful combination of ventricular tachycardia followed by ventricular flutter and ventricular fibrillation and he died.

Review Tracing 49

This is a condition of Ashman phenomenon. The E.C.G. shows sinus bradycardia interrupted by runs of supraventricular ectopic beats giving the appearance of pulsus trigeminus at times. Slower the heart rate, longer the refractory period of the heart, the nodal beat falling within the refractory period of the preceding QRS complex which has followed a long R-R interval, has an aberrant ventricular conduction; the nodal beat is immediatly followed by another atrial ectopic beat; the tripled beats are thus constituted by a sinus beat, a nodal ectopic beat and an atrial ectopic beat.

Review Tracing 50

Av. ht. rate 81/min. Sinus rhythm, normal axis, vertical lie, early infarction inferior wall.

Review Tracing 51

Av. ht. rate 72/mn. Sinus rhythm, Normal axis, Intermediate lie, myocardial infarction of some duration antero-septal & lat wall.

Review Tracing 52

Av. ht. rate 45/min, Sinus rhythm, Normal axis, Intermediate lie, Rt bundle branch block pattern, 2:1 heart block intermittently with complete heart block, Ischaemic changes septal wall.

Review Tracing 53

Av. ht. rate 88/min, Sinus rhythm intercepted by supraventricular ectopics of multicentric origin with aberrant conduction, left axis, horizontal lie, Incomplete rt. bundle branch block, marked clockwise rotation which may be due to old anteroseptal and lateral wall infarction, Ischaemia inferolat. wall.

Review Tracing 54

Av. heart rate 162/min, Supraventricular tachycardia possibly nodal, normal axis, Intermediate lie, diffuse myocardial ischaemia, right bundle branch block.

Review Tracing 55

Av. heart rate 98/min, Sinus rhythm intercepted by single and runs of nodal ectopics with occasional nodal escape beats semivertical lie, Intermittent aberrant conduction, right bundle branch block.

INDEX

Figures in the parentheses indicate page numbers of the illustrative tracings.